Living Life to the Full: My Ironman Journey

From open-heart surgery to an Ironman triathlon in just eight months

Ellen Charnley

First published by Dog Ear Publishing
4010 W. 86th Street, Ste H
Indianapolis, IN 46268
www.dogearpublishing.net

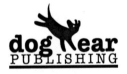

ISBN: 978-145750-122-7

This book is printed on acid-free paper.

Printed in the United States of America

ACKNOWLEDGMENTS

I started writing this memoir on the flight home to Vegas from the Cleveland Clinic hospital. This was one week after my open-heart surgery. I wrote the details that I could remember at the time about the surgery and the events leading up to it, to ensure that I would never forget them or my emotions and actions. I wanted to remember so I would never take my experiences for granted and so someday I would be able to open this memoir and appreciate all that happened. In those early days of writing, I had no intention—or, frankly, any notion—of turning my scribbles into a published memoir, and only after having lighthearted discussions with friends did I come to the conclusion that perhaps just maybe some folks might find this interesting and even possibly a motivational read. With that in mind, I continued to write and have enjoyed the process tremendously. It has been extremely therapeutic and at times oddly revealing to me, especially as I have dug deep into my inner thoughts and early life experiences. I have shared with you my feelings and emotions; everything written is the truth, and I have written this, of course, from my heart.

Thank you to all of my friends both in Vegas and afar who provided me with the physical and mental support during the spring of 2010; without this support, getting to the right decisions would have been so much harder. Camilla, thank you for taking the time to write the Foreword to my memoir. You have an amazing ability to listen and to provide unconditional support, love, and loyalty. You will always be a true friend.

Dougal, Amy, and Bob, thank you for being such dedicated and motivational training partners throughout the summer of 2010. Thank you for always looking back to make sure I was behind you. To my swim coach, Paul, thank you for pushing me and helping me to realize I could actually swim fast at age 41!

Thank you also to my brother, Paul, for your counsel and guiding words of logic and reason. You have always been there for me, and for that I am truly grateful. To my parents, thank you for understanding my decision not to tell you until after the surgery.

Thank you to the wonderful team at the Cleveland Clinic. You are all incredibly talented, and without your attention to detail, I doubt I would be here to write this memoir. To my primary care physician, your thoroughness and determination to get the correct diagnosis helped save my life. Thank you to my cardiologist at the University of Washington. You provided me with the final support and direction that I needed to get to the starting line of the Ironman, and you truly do understand my passion.

If you are searching for inspiration or motivation to take on a challenge, then I hope you succeed, however large or small the challenge may be. I also hope that you consider adopting the advice that my husband instilled in me more than twenty-three years ago and that I now follow every single moment of every single day… that you live life to the full. Don, to you, I am forever grateful for your inspiration, motivation, and love for all of my adult life and for providing me with the strength to embrace this past year's challenges. You are my hero, my soul mate, and I love you dearly.

FOREWORD

I first met Ellen at a Sprint Triathlon at Lake Mead, Las Vegas, in 2009. She and Don had persuaded my husband that it would be a "fun little competition," and he was duly enticed. As I stood watching the triathletes jostle their way through the water, I noticed that it was a relatively small female who was the first to touch dry land. Not only was she in the lead, but she had managed to make the swim look effortless and ran into the transition area minutes ahead of her competitors. I watched her as she leapt onto her bike with a sense of balance I knew to be foreign to the average bystander, and I was intrigued to see that despite finishing the bike ride strong and unfazed, and comfortably on the leaders' board, she didn't attempt the run.

I was later introduced to Ellen Charnley, pre-knee surgery, pre-heart surgery.

This book is about an extraordinary woman who, despite rising odds and both physical and emotional setbacks, never lost sight of her goal to complete one of the most grueling feats of athleticism. But Ellen's story isn't that simple. Not only did she overcome health hurdles of the highest magnitude, but she managed to keep her high-powered job, marriage, and friendships blooming; no simple feat when forced to confront life at its core.

These past eight months of Ellen's life define the true meaning of "inspirational." When forced to adjust her way of living, she refused to adjust her dreams. She displays the essence of the human spirit in its most determined and most courageous form, and above all, she does so with an unwavering strength of sheer will power.

Camilla Beevor, December 2010

CHAPTER ONE

ICU

I open my eyes, and the sense of relief is overwhelming, just to wake up and know that my heart did, after all, "restart." This had preyed on my mind ever since I had been told that during open-heart surgery, my heart would be stopped and my body would continue to survive via a heart-lung machine.

Once the novelty of the relief wears off, next comes the pain—not from my chest but rather my throat and back. I feel a tube in my throat. I can't swallow. I am desperately thirsty. The tube is connected to a machine that helps me to breathe. Nurses swarm around me as I awaken, reassuring me constantly that everything is normal and that the surgery has gone well. They tell me that I have to be patient (now I know where the word comes from) and gradually start to breathe more on my own. Eventually, when I can prove I am doing so unassisted, they will remove the tube.

I move my head and start to register where I am. The intensive care unit, the Cleveland Clinic, March 26, 2010. I am in a bed that is separated from other patient beds by only a curtain. The room seems large, but I have no real perception. There is lots of activity happening, nurses attending to patients, but I can see very little, as my vision is limited to the space immediately in front of my bed, where I see a specialized nurses' station positioned with a nurse sitting there, just a few feet away from me.

Don arrives shortly after I awake; he's been waiting patiently for six hours. The Cleveland Clinic has a system for open-heart surgery patients and their families; it's tried and tested day after day, year after year for thousands of patients. The Cleveland Clinic is a reassuring place—well, as reassuring as any cardiac surgical hospital can be.

I subsequently learn from Don that once the surgery was completed, my surgeon had left the operating room and greeted Don in the family waiting area. He had told Don that the surgery was a success. At this time, he had also informed Don that my condition had been far worse than they had originally thought and that the previously counted four holes in my heart were now "numerous" and too many to count. The medical term to describe the wall of my defective heart was "Swiss cheese." Surgery had most definitely been the only option. He used descriptive phrases such as "wet tissue paper" to describe the weakened wall structure. He also explained that the right side of my heart was three times the size of the left. Given this, he told Don that it was questionable how much longer my heart would have been able to keep functioning, regardless of whether I continued to push my body competitively training and racing triathlon. After the procedure had been carried out and the holes repaired, the surgeon claimed, the right side of the heart had immediately begun to reduce in size.

Every designated family member carries a pager so they can be quickly contacted during the hours after surgery. Two hours after meeting my surgeon, Don was paged in the "family waiting" area and was able to come to my bedside. That's how long it took to close me up and go through the finishing touches of the surgery. By approximately 8:00 p.m., seven hours after I had said good-bye and he had wished me good luck, he began his new role of coach as he helped me through the next few hours of misery.

The sense of fear is quite overwhelming, and time moves very slowly. The nurses gather around my bed and begin asking me to perform some simple tasks. "Ellen, can you wiggle your toes for me?" I oblige. "Ellen, now squeeze my hand." Again, I oblige. Don and the nurses begin to ask me questions that require simple "yes" or "no" gestures, as I am unable to speak because of the tube restriction. "Ellen, are you in pain?" I nod. The nurses increase my pain medication, a quick process, as the morphine-related drug is administered directly into the IV in my neck, the central line. I feel a little relief instantly.

I start to feel the need to ask questions, so the communication method soon progresses and I begin to spell out the first letter of each word on my hand, at the suggestion of the nurse. I write on her palm. This continues slowly. I point to the tube in my mouth and motion that I want the nurse to remove it. She shakes her head and tells me we have a little while longer to wait. I am becoming more stressed; I hear my monitors start to bleep as my heart rate falls. I motion with my hand that I want to write my questions with a pen and paper. I cannot lift my head or really move my arms to a great extent, so my writing skills are very limited. Don and the nurses do extremely well to interpret my words, although to I, lying flat on my back and heavily sedated, I feel my writing skills are near perfection. I've since seen these scribbles and now feel that Don and I can challenge anyone at Pictionary and win hands down. The specifics of these "conversations" are at best a blur now, but I know that they revolved around me continually asking how much longer I had to wait before they would remove the tube.

Don places the ear bud from my iPod into my right ear and sets the music to some soft tune in an attempt to calm my fear momentarily. At the time my music of choice was from the singer-song writer David Gray, whom we had, coincidentally, seen live only a week before in Cleveland. David Gray's album *Draw the Line* helped me through those first few days and will forever bring back those memories.

I hold Don's hand and do not let go. Finally, the moment has arrived; a nurse explains that they are going to remove the tube. What a great achievement. I'm very excited. I later learned that a patient begins to assess his or her progress by monitoring how many tubes, monitors, IVs, and pipes are still inserted and how many are being removed during each day in hospital. When all of these are removed, there is a hope that the patient can be discharged. The removal of the breathing tube for me now is step one on the road to recovery. Two nurses crowd close to me; one monitors, the other explains that they will pull the inner tube first by simply pulling it from deep down in my stomach. I am asked to relax. It hurts down into my back and throat as they pull. This inner tube is performing some role in my stomach. Next, they slowly tug at the outer tube. As they pull gently, I am asked to cough. I also begin to gag, but within seconds, the tube is out and I am asked to state my name and birth date and where I am. "Ellen Charnley, March 6,

1969, Cleveland Clinic." They ask why I am here. "I had heart surgery to fix some holes." The sound of my voice is weak and a few notches higher than normal, as if I've inhaled some helium from a party balloon, but that soon wears off. The pain is less now.

I am now able to speak. I ask Don about his meeting with my surgeon. My blood pressure and heart rate are very low. I ask the nurses about this; they are not concerned and again reassure me. I am sleepy but am scared to sleep. What if I don't awaken again? More drugs are given to me to numb the pain, which is centered on the right side of my chest and back. I am desperately thirsty. The nurse brings a plastic cup full of ice chips. I cannot reach the cup holder, so the nurse gently lifts my head and places a spoon of ice chips into my mouth. She tells me I cannot have more than one spoon this time around, my stomach needs to wake up from the surgery, too, and that will take time. The ice melts quickly in my mouth, and the water drips down my throat, a heavenly moment amidst the chaos running through my brain and body. The nurse places the cup of ice purposely out of my reach and tells me she will let me have more in a short while. I want to gulp a full glass of water or, better still, orange juice. I haven't drunk a drop for close to 20 hours. The saline that has been pumped into my body during this time has hydrated my body but has done nothing for my thirst.

Around midnight, Don prepares to leave for the hotel room and some much-needed sleep. I let go of his hand and make him promise he will be back when I wake in a few hours. The nurses tell him they will call him around 8 a.m. after the morning rounds are over. While back in his hotel room, before he goes to bed, he dutifully e-mails our friends and family with an update on my condition. I begin my first night in the ICU—the intensive care unit. I am a triathlete; I am healthy and very fit. It is hard to comprehend that I am currently incapacitated and in the ICU.

 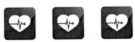

I had watched the "What to Expect" video the day before surgery, and frankly, this scared me, seeing a patient lying in her bed in the ICU, hooked up to numerous monitors and the breathing tube. This was a tough day for me mentally, anticipating, fearing, and trying hard to stay focused on positives rather than the what-ifs. For most people, open-heart surgery isn't on their bucket list, and I would certainly recommend avoiding it if you have the option. As a consequence, few people know much about it and what to expect. For example, until the day before my surgery, I didn't know that to operate on my heart, they would stop it beating first. To do this, they would use the heart-lung machine, clamp the aorta, and use medication to stop my heart from beating. This is a pretty frightening thing to learn the day before surgery.

The more I learned, the more I feared. I started to believe that I still had a choice, that somehow, my heart would miraculously function just fine for another 40 or 50 years and I would still complete my Ironman triathlon dream. I came close to backing out; it was open-heart surgery, after all, and it just wasn't on my agenda at age 41.

I think the reality hit during the meeting with my surgeon the day before. He simply told me the facts—compassionately, but still, they were the facts. He said I no longer had a choice and the procedure was not "elective" but urgent and that without the surgery, my heart would undoubtedly fail. Tears began to roll down my face as the fear started to creep in. These words hit home and helped me mentally get to where I needed to be. At that moment I started to move from denial, where I had been for the past three days, to acceptance. But with acceptance came overwhelming fear.

It is now past midnight, and I am scared to see him go but so high from the medication, I don't fight his departure too much, and I understand he needs to rest and most likely to leave the ICU just for a few hours. I am breathing on my own. The nurses' shift changes over, and my new caregiver takes her position at the end of my bed. David Gray is still quietly singing in my ear. The right side of my chest and back hurt from the pain.

There are no glass sliding doors in this ICU. It is not like I had imagined from watching TV hospital dramas. There are no quarantined sections, just a ward full of beds, nurses, patients, and complicated equipment. The sounds consist of monitors beeping, alarms ringing, and occasional Code Blue announcements over the loudspeaker. ICU is not a quiet place. The nurses are giving the patients instructions, particularly on what not to do. I hear a patient groaning two beds down from mine. The nurses are telling him to stop biting the breathing tube. I suspect he is in pain and doesn't realize he is biting the tube. The nurses keep at him to stop and don't remove the tube; they talk to each other as if he cannot hear them. His name is Daniel.

ICU nurses are nurses at the top of their field. They are well respected and have trained and worked hard to get to this position. I cannot imagine doing their job, having patients' lives in my hands day in day out.

The night ticks on, lots going on, I drift in and out of a sleepy haze. The noises wake me. New nurses arrive; one of them is responsible for making me breath into a breathing tube. I have to breathe hard enough to get the line above the blue marker. I try hard and achieve this on the first attempt. I am pleased; one more step to recovery. After the breathing, he asks me to cough hard, but when I cough, it hurts, and my chest feels ready to explode. I cough up thick mucus as my lungs begin to clear; I am told this is normal and what they want me to continue to do. A different nurse constantly monitors and charts my vital signs; she is with me every minute, and I am reassured. A central venous pressure line has been inserted in my left arm and connects to their vital-sign monitor so my blood pressure and heartbeat are constantly monitored. This is why this area is called the intensive care unit. The care you receive is simply full-on 100-percent intensive.

Two or three times during the night, I panic as I doze; my heart rate and blood pressure drop again and my alarms ring. My anxiety and fear rise, which makes things worse, and my pain increases. As I am an avid triathlete, my blood pressure and resting heart rate are typically below the average Joe's. My history and athletic achievements are known to the nurses, so they are not concerned with the alarms ringing. I am still concerned, though, as I know that the readings are now below what is normal for even me. I am scared to sleep, and I tell my nurse, Courtney, this. She reassures me that everything is normal and they are watching me; she holds my hand and strokes my forehead and tells me to sleep. I am cold, so she brings me another blanket. The temperature in the hospital is purposely kept cold, especially in the ICU.

The heart takes a beating during surgery and takes a short while to get its groove back, so during most heart surgeries, thin wires are placed into the heart and threaded out through the skin in the chest. If necessary, these wires are then connected to a machine, which can regulate the heart rate and give it a helping hand. The nurses attach my wires to this device, and this increases my heart rate to an acceptable level. This eases my anxiety, and I fall asleep. Every time I wake, my nurse reassures me that everything is normal and I am doing great. The nurses all spend a large proportion of their time with me performing this function. On more than one occasion, tears start to fall down my face; I am still scared. I had open-heart surgery; what if something goes wrong?

At this time, I don't understand all the different pain, and the days that follow will all add to my pain education and help reduce my fear. I am on some serious medication in the ICU, all of it fed through my central IV line, which is located in my neck. I don't feel the needles in my neck but do feel the cool liquids flushing into my body. I also have another IV in my right arm, and one in my hand, although I'm not sure what these are used for.

Saline is the doctors' favorite liquid. The first IV that someone receives before surgery contains nothing but saline, and it is given in the pre-op room before the patient heads into the OR. That was when I first experienced the "saline sensation." Almost immediately, the taste of the saline ended up in my mouth. I learn to tolerate this taste, as I am to experience it numerous times each day for the next week. With this sensation comes weight gain and a bloating throughout the entire body. I was 130 lbs the morning before the surgery. Six days later, after having eaten very little, vomited three times, and experienced an afternoon of diarrhea, I was 137 lbs. What kind of justice is that! Water retention is a hazard of surgery, as the body is pumped full of salt.

 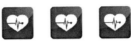

Five months earlier, I had completed in two-thirds of a full Ironman triathlon on one of the tenth most difficult courses in the world as ranked by *Triathlete* magazine: the Silverman Triathlon, Las Vegas, Nevada, 2009. I swam 2.4 miles and rode 112 miles through a steep, hilly terrain in the desert, the last 35 miles of which I did with sight from only one of my eyes. This made depth perception a little challenging. I had been suffering from temporary blurred vision during my long training rides and had somewhat put this to the back of my mind until after the race, simply putting it down to the dry Vegas air or an issue with my contact lens.

A knee injury had plagued me all year and had sidelined my running training from April 2009 through the rest of the year, so swimming and biking had become my focus. By focusing on these two disciplines, I had been able to really push myself and achieve results that were pretty damn good for me. I had hired a coach who pushed me to my limits on the swim, bringing back many childhood memories along the way. The two highlights of that summer were coming in second overall in the aquabike division at the Vineman Half Ironman distance and then completing the Silverman with a 59-minute, 2.4-mile swim. It was a season of personal bests. I had trained, raced, and achieved these results with multiple holes in my heart that were unknown to me at the time.

Following the Silverman race, I had scheduled knee surgery to have my left knee scoped after nine months of delibera-tion, physical therapy, and cortisone shots. I had the surgery in November 2009, the plan being that I would then have the winter, or "off-season," to recover before I would begin training for Ironman Arizona, which would be in November 2010. Completing a full Ironman has long been my dream:

swimming 2.4 miles, biking 112 miles, and running a full 26.2-mile marathon, continuously. In November 2009, I successfully registered online for the race, a full year in advance and just two weeks after my knee surgery. Ironman racing has become so popular in recent years that a race can sell out online within minutes of it becoming available. I paid my $550 entrance fee and was excited about the year ahead and the journey to realizing my dream.

I awake during the night, Courtney gives me another delicious spoonful of ice chips, and in return I have to promise another round of breathing exercises. One more breath into my breathing device would make it 10 in a row that I had breathed hard enough to raise the blue marker above the required line. One more step to recovery. One more step to my Ironman goal.

At 8:00 a.m. on March 27, 2010, one day post surgery, I notice the clock on the wall above the foot of my bed. The phone rings, and my nurse answers; it is Don checking in. He tells her he will come over to the ICU around 9:30 a.m. I don't remember sleeping, but I must have, as I can't account for the past few hours of the early morning. More monitoring and more medication. I am now able to reach the ice chips myself. What freedom. My mouth thinks it's won the lottery, but I am cautioned by my morning nurse not to overdo it.

Don arrives at 9:30 a.m. and sits with me and takes hold of my hand. I had never realized the value of human touch during times of stress until this moment. I tell him about my pain and my night. He seems simply happy or relieved, I'm not sure which, but calm; as usual, he shows no concern, which is what I need to see.

My next visitor is my surgeon. It is a Saturday and not normally a day he would be working in the hospital, but he is on his way to the airport for a well-deserved vacation. He stops by my bed to see me. He repeats the conversation that he had with Don the previous day, telling me that the operation was a success and that my road to recovery will be quick.

He also confirms that the surgery was most definitely the only viable option for treatment. I tell him I have pain in the right side of my chest, and he explains this is most likely from the chest tube that was inserted during surgery and is planned for removal today before I leave the ICU. The chest tube is a drainage pipe that comes out of an incision in the skin on the chest and drains all the unnecessary posttraumatic fluids that the body accumulates, thus preventing infections by draining. Thankfully, I can't see the tube or the contents of the drainage pack.

Don offers to fetch me a fruit popsicle from the ICU kitchen. He brings me a grape-flavored one, and it tastes heavenly. Time ticks on, and finally, I hear discussions about me leaving the ICU today. It is 2:00 p.m. If all continues to go well, I am to be transferred to a step-down ward later this afternoon. I am one step closer to recovery, but my feelings are not of relief but apprehension. The nursing attention in the step-down ward will be less intensive, and that fills me with more fear. Each step-down ward has one nurse to five or six patients.

I've never been admitted to a hospital before, excluding the outpatient knee surgery the previous November, and hospitals have always frightened me. I remember that during my childhood, our family always seemed to be overly concerned about illness, to the extent that during my teenage years, I was at times arguably a borderline hypochondriac. That was before I met Don during the first year at university, age 18. Don's view on illness is the complete opposite; he always denies having a cold, believes illness can be controlled by the mind to a large degree, and never, ever looks on the pessimistic side of things. I have never encountered anyone more positive. What better person to partner with me for the rest of my life and teach me the value of positive thinking and its power over healing? Now in the ICU as I deal with pain I have never experienced before, Don helps me visualize my "happy place" and focus on my positive thinking.

My happy place is part of the virtual imagery session we went through in the pre-op process. I was asked to imagine a place where I would feel safe and happy and could heal with my family and friends around me. For me, this place was simple to find. The image has always been the same, but until the pre-op imagery session, I had never realized or visualized where it was. Perhaps this place is heaven; I'm happy thinking

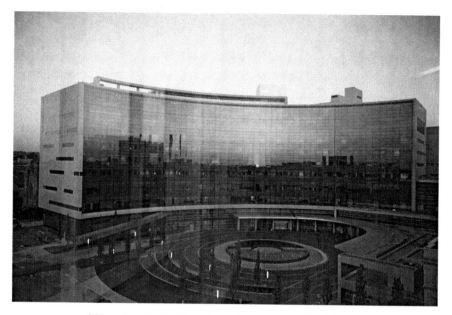

Miller Family Pavilion Heart Center, Cleveland Clinic

that. My heaven is a large oak tree on the top of an English hilltop in the countryside, always with the sun shining and many rabbits playing at the foot of the tree, their home. Don helps me focus on my happy place when the pain and discomfort grow.

I am still in pain, particularly in my right side, where the chest tube is. My current nurse tells me it's time to remove the tube. I thank God. Another nurse assists her during the process. They begin first by giving me more medication, and I instantly feel drowsy. They lift my right arm and unbutton my hospital gown, exposing most of the right side of my body. They gently peel away at the bandages that are stuck to my skin. They then firmly pull the tube out from the incision in my chest. I feel the tugging sensation, but the pain is masked by the medication. They leave the wound open without bandaging it again; it already has two or three stitches to hold the incision together. While my gown is open, the nurse inspects my main scar. This is underneath my right breast. I am not able to see it myself, but she tells me it is healing nicely. Don takes a look and seems surprised and impressed with the neatness and skill of the doctors and nurses who closed me up.

A few more hours pass. Transportation arrives as I am about to begin my journey to the step-down ward and be discharged from the ICU, just 24 hours after my arrival. I am assisted into a wheelchair; my head spins, my legs have no strength, and I rely heavily on the nurses to support me. They tell me to use the strength in my quads and take the weight if I can. I am a long way from walking, let alone running. I am wheeled to my step-down ward, J5-3, room 4.

CHAPTER TWO

Step-Down, J5-3, Room 4.

March 2010

I am in J5-3, floor 5 of the new cardiac unit, area 3, room 4. This is a step-down ward for recovering heart-surgery patients. It will be my home for the next few days. The Cleveland Clinic is no ordinary hospital, and I am truly fortunate to be a patient here. My private room is akin to a room in a five-star hotel: flat-screen TV, en-suite bathroom, and chic (but apparently uncomfortable) pull-out couch for a family member to sleep on. There are no restrictions to visiting hours, and loved ones are welcome 24 hours a day. The patient beds are very high-tech; every possible angle and position is available to make the patient more comfortable at the touch of button.

On Saturday afternoon at 4:00 p.m., Linda is my first nurse on the floor. She greets me and chats with the transportation team and the nurse who accompanied them from the ICU. I am wheeled into my new room, and even though I am struggling to keep my head up, I take a look around and marvel at the room's size, cleanliness, and technology. In the days leading up to the surgery, I wondered if I would be fortunate enough to occupy my own room. Once again, my perspective has dramatically changed. At this moment, all I want to do is lie down again and get out of the wheelchair. There could be 20 patients crammed into this tiny ward for all I care at this moment.

Linda's first role is to assist me from the wheelchair to the bed in the center of the room. She politely tells me to stand momentarily before moving backwards onto the bed. I hold onto the two transport team members as I try to take more weight with my quads. I start to tremble, and the transporters tighten their grip. I am shocked at my lack of strength; just a few days ago, I was running for six miles around the park in Cleveland. Linda tells me she has to inspect my behind. She gives no reason why, and I don't ask; I presume she is checking for bedsores. I am no longer embarrassed; I don't care. I feel nauseated and need to lie down to stop my head spinning. Satisfied with her inspection, Linda lowers my gown and indicates that I am allowed to move backward to the bed and carefully lower myself back. Linda's next task is to hook me back up to the monitors and to take vital signs. She also reconnects my IV. I'm exhausted, and the pain meds make me drowsy. The journey was little more than a few hundred yards from the ICU, but I feel like I have completed a triathlon.

 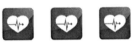

I learned of my heart defect on March 2. The decisions and conversations that took place during those three weeks between discovery and the surgery were intense and occupied my mind like nothing else ever has. I learned that my mind works in very interesting ways; what is important at one point seems somewhat irrelevant a moment later. Training for an Ironman was my focus following my knee surgery, and I had begun a structured training program from January, building up all three disciplines, swimming, biking, and running slowly but very surely. This was my base training period. Training for the Ironman still dominated my thoughts as I visited the Cleveland Clinic that first week in March, and I was simply frustrated at the time that I could not adequately train that week or the week following as I recovered from a battery of medical testing.

I had been referred to the clinic in January after seeing my local primary care physician in Las Vegas. My bike-riding blindness had caused her some concern, and she felt this blindness was caused by something wrong either with my eye or, worse, the blood supply getting to my eye. She first referred me to an ophthalmologist the very next day. I had two thorough examinations with him, and he concluded that my eye was completely normal and the temporary vision loss had not damaged it in any way. I guessed this was good news, although the question as to what was causing the blindness was becoming more difficult to answer. The ophthalmologist ordered a brain MRI to "rule out anything nasty." I never questioned him about this, but I presumed he was referring to a brain tumor or something equally frightening. I felt fine and, because of my knee surgery, had not been doing any long bike rides, so I was almost happy convincing myself that whatever the problem was, it was unlikely to still be evident.

The MRI didn't reveal anything of interest, but the radiologist suggested to the doctor that I undergo a head CT, as this would look more closely at the arteries and blood vessels in my head. On December 23, 2009, I had a follow up appointment with my primary care physician to discuss the results of this latest test. Evidently, I had something abnormal in my right ophthalmic artery, a "beading" and "narrowness." My doctor was concerned about vascular disease yet admitted that she was no expert on the subject. She kindly told me to wait while she spoke with a local neurologist. The neurologist apparently directed her to a doctor who specializes in cerebral vasculitis. This doctor was located at the Cleveland Clinic.

Within a few days, I received a call from this doctor at the Cleveland Clinic, who chatted through some of the possible causes of my test result. He strongly advised that I visit the hospital for a week of testing, in particular to undergo a cerebral angiogram, the apparent gold standard of all brain tests. He ended our conversation by asking me if I had concerns or was worried about anything; this was after he had explained some possible theories behind my condition, none of which were too pleasant, such as cerebral vasculitis, fibromuscular dysplasia, or multiple sclerosis. At the time I thought this was an odd question; of course I was concerned. But looking back, I realize I was probably still just a little irritated that this was going to disrupt my training plans.

We arrived at the clinic on March 1, and I began a week of invasive testing and specialist appointments from early in the morning until early evening every day. I was physically and mentally exhausted. During that week, I had 16 tubes of blood drawn; ultrasounds of my eye, carotid arteries, renal arteries, and heart; a 90-minute, very claustrophobic, MRI of my midsection while I held my breath every minute; physical examinations by an eye doctor, a vascular specialist, a neurologist, a cardiologist, and all their accompanying nurses and resident doctors; an MRI of the brain; a transesophageal echocardiogram; my eyes dilated; and a cerebral angiogram. Not all of these tests had originally been planned but rather evolved the more the doctors looked further into my case. The gold-standard cerebral angiogram was scheduled for Tuesday 2 March and required that I be admitted to the hospital radiology department for a day.

We were instructed to arrive in the radiology department in the basement of the hospital, H1-B. Of course I was not allowed to eat or drink anything before the procedure, so to spare me the pain of smelling the piping-hot freshly brewed Starbucks coffee, Don took a detour on his own to purchase his morning cup. As I checked into the front desk, I was rudely asked where my "family member" was and who was going to drive me home that evening. At this point I wasn't really aware of what the test involved, but I kindly explained to the woman at the desk that my husband would wheel me back to my hotel room if I was unable to walk. I was given a pager and told to wait in the waiting room. Don arrived back and waited patiently with me until the nurse called my name. We followed the nurse through the double doors into the pre-op waiting room. I was shown to a bed, and the nurse politely asked me to undress, drawing the curtain to give me some privacy. Next, my vital signs were taken and I was asked to explain my understanding of the procedure. I think I did a fairly decent job, but clearly, she was not impressed, so before long, a doctor arrived at my bed and explained in more detail what was going to happen. He also shared with me the risks, the most important one being that the test could trigger a stroke, although that was unlikely. He asked if I still wished to continue. I didn't really feel I had a choice.

I had a few more hours of waiting before I was finally escorted to the operating room. Several nurses and doctors were milling around. The room was incredibly cold, and I shivered violently. One of the nurses seemed concerned about this and covered me in additional blankets. They started an IV and hooked me up to a machine to monitor my vital signs. Another nurse checked to see if I was completely naked and joked that the previous patient had arrived wearing underwear and the doctors had been none too happy with the nurses because of it. Two doctors arrived into the room and explained that the procedure was going to begin. One injected a local anesthetic into my groin and then cut an opening in my groin. I was given a light sedation and began to feel drowsy. Next, a probe was inserted through the opening in my groin into the femoral artery and up into my brain. I was awake the entire time and was able to hold my breath and answer questions when asked. The test did not hurt, with the exception of the incision in my groin.

During the test, I learned that, despite an abnormal CT scan in Las Vegas, the angiogram had come back negative. This was extremely surprising to everyone at the clinic and to me. My arteries were normal, with no narrowing or beading and therefore no answer to my vision issues. I became irritated that the test had almost been a waste of time, and this irritation was increased when I learned that I had to spend the next six hours in a short-stay hospital ward and lie completely flat during this time to ensure that the femoral artery did not bleed out and could clot properly. I should have felt relief that the angiogram was negative, but I felt frustrated that we were no further in finding an answer to my blindness. I was transported to the short-stay ward and greeted by the head nurse. I remember thinking that she was kind, my first real experience of a hospital nurse. She instructed me that under no circumstances could I lift my head, body, or legs; I was to lie completely flat. She inspected my groin and checked for bleeding. It was fine. I had to lie there for six hours. After four hours, I started to fantasize about urinating. My bladder was getting full, and I knew I couldn't hold on for another two hours. I called the nurse, and she gave me a bedpan. This was my first humbling experience at the hospital. For women, a bedpan is very cumbersome.

Through all these tests, we had successfully ruled out some fairly nasty diseases, so there was definite cause for some celebration, but even the "Dr. House" of the Cleveland Clinic was unable to conclusively say why I was losing my vision in my right eye. During that six-hour hospital stay, however, I learned of my heart condition.

I was dreaming of coffee and so sent Don off to Starbucks to purchase me one. Soon after he had left the ward, my bedside phone rang. It was the vascular medicine doctor. She was calling to inform me that my heart echocardiogram was abnormal. I had met with this specialist the day before for an extensive physical exam, during which she had heard a murmur in my heart through her stethoscope. For 41 years, doctors have listened to my heart, but no one else had ever heard this murmur. By fortunate coincidence, this doctor was also a trained cardiologist, and one of her specialties was training medical interns how to detect heart murmurs. On hearing my murmur, she had immediately ordered an echo of my heart that day. During the call, she calmly told me that something was wrong with my heart, a condition that I had had since birth, and that she had been able to get me an appointment with the director of the Adult Congenital Heart Disease program at the clinic the following morning. At this time, I was becoming somewhat immune to the tests and examinations, so having one more doctor to see didn't significantly concern me at this point. I wasn't aware at this time, however, how serious my condition was. She also recommended that Don and I should delay our departure from Cleveland and if possible postpone our flights, as it was likely there were more tests in store.

A congenital condition is a condition someone is born with. According to the Adult Congenital Heart Association, approximately one million adults and 800,000 children are living with congenital heart defects in the United States. At least 10% of all congenital heart defects are first found in adulthood, as was the case with me. Many adults do not have symptoms from these defects until age 30 or 40. Common long-term problems include enlargement of the right side of the heart, rhythm problems, valve problems, heart failure, heart infection, and stroke. Many adults require surgery to fix their defects. Virtually all adults who live beyond the age of 60 with congenital heart defects become symptomatic, and if their condition is left untreated, the average survival rate beyond 40 or 50 years is 50%.

In the space of an hour that next morning, I was quickly educated on my specific defects. Atrial septal defects (ASDs) are holes in the septum (wall) between the top atria (upper chambers). ASDs account for approximately 7% of all congenital heart defects and are three times more likely in women than in men. According to my echocardiogram (heart ultrasound) the previous day, I had two or possibly three of these holes of varying sizes and a very flimsy-looking septum as a consequence (medically termed an aneurism). In addition, the right side of my heart was severely enlarged. The doctor explained that there was a strong likelihood that he could fix these holes percutaneously (that is, by using a very thin catheter via the femoral artery, in a process similar to the angiogram procedure that I had undergone the day before) by placing a small device into the wall to plug the holes. To be sure, however, he needed me to undergo another test, a transesophageal echocardiogram, or TEE, a rather unpleasant test in which, under moderate sedation and a throat-numbing medicine, I would have an ultrasound probe inserted down my throat to take pictures of my heart behind my ribcage. This procedure provides a clearer view than the above-surface echo. I was becoming immune to the barrage of tests that were being scheduled and was just grateful that all of this was being taken care of promptly so I could resume training as quickly as possible.

The TEE was scheduled for the following day and was the most unpleasant test I had ever experienced. The sedation was not strong enough, and my gag reflux was difficult to control. I was once again in a hospital gown, lying on a bed, with another IV. During the procedure, the doctors looked at the images that the probe projected onto the screen, and even though I was sedated, I remember distinctly their surprised tone as they examined the findings. The TEE revealed a worse picture than they had previously thought, with at least three or possibly more holes, one significantly large (1.5 cm in diameter), and all, unfortunately, spread far apart across the wall. The test itself lasted a couple of hours, but in total, I was back in a hospital bed for almost half a day. My cardiologist had also come down to the lab when I was having the test performed to see the results on screen in real time. The pain was very unpleasant, and this must have become clear to the nurse and the doctor, as he instructed her to increase the medication to make me more relaxed. Still, I heard their conversation and understood that the results were not great. Finally, they finished and the nurse pulled out the tube at the same time as I coughed. I was then wheeled back to a recovery ward, and after an hour, my cardiologist visited my bedside. He told me the condition was worse than they had first thought and that for a complete fix, I should consider open-heart surgery. This was the first mention of surgery, and instantly, I dismissed this option. He explained, however, that he was willing to attempt to fix the holes percutaneously if that was the decision I wanted to make.

Lying back in my bed, I realize my newfound stomachache is actually my menstrual cycle beginning, early for my inconvenience, apparently a classic side effect of stress. I have a urinary catheter inserted and am attached to a bag that drains the catheter with my urine. I never have the urge to pee, which, given that I can't get to the bathroom, is a relief. I am not wearing underwear because of the catheter, however, so I am leaking blood onto the bed. I tell Linda in an apologetic tone when she is next in my room. She looks at me sweetly and helps me move into a different position while she lays down protective sheets. She then helps me to a standing position, and helplessly, I hold onto her shoulders as she carefully bathes me, working around the catheter. Another very humbling moment. I ask Linda what she tells her husband when she goes home at night; she laughs and says she is here to take care of me and nothing really fazes her. I feel a connection with Linda and am grateful she is my nurse.

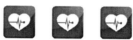

After they discovered my congenital heart defects, we scheduled the percutaneous procedure for March 22 with my cardiologist, although the exact nature of the procedure at this point was still a little unclear. My cardiologist was reasonably confident that he could perform a partial fix by this method and insert one, maybe two, occlusion devices (synthetic small mesh devices that plug the holes in the heart wall); however, his recommendation even at this stage was surgery for a 100% fix. He was concerned that the defects were too numerous, large, and far apart to be fixed percutaneously. He was also concerned that only fixing part of the defects may not solve the vision issues that I was having. I discussed these issues with him on two occasions during the two weeks that followed while Don and I were back in Vegas. I continually resisted the surgical option, and my cardiologist and I agreed to move forward with the less-than-perfect percutaneous solution. Even if it was only a partial fix, it was good enough, right? Wrong.

We flew back to Cleveland on Saturday, March 20 and tried to enjoy the weekend, running and relaxing. On Sunday morning, we saw an advertisement for singer-song writer David Gray playing for a one-night-only concert in Cleveland that evening. David Gray is one of my favorite music artists, so we called the box office. Call it fortune or fate, but we purchased the last two tickets for the concert. It was a fabulous event.

I met with my cardiologist on Monday morning and also had more blood drawn. We discussed the plan for the following day.

On March 23, the day of my scheduled percutaneous procedure, I arrived at 9:00 a.m. and was immediately assigned a bed and cubicle and asked to undress and don the now all-too-familiar Cleveland Clinic gown. A nurse took my vital signs and demanded a urine sample to confirm I wasn't pregnant. Doctors and nurses never believe the patients! Finally, both sides of my groin were shaved, and then I waited. Don was paged to come to my bedside. Together, we waited and waited. Some time later, a doctor appeared at my bedside and introduced himself as an interventional cardiologist working in the cath lab. This is a division of doctors that perform these less invasive catheter-style procedures rather than surgery. He was unknown to me but appeared to know much about me and my condition. He explained that he wasn't convinced that the percutaneous treatment would be successful, and he almost insisted that I at least see a surgeon before I underwent the percutaneous procedure to get a surgical opinion, as in his opinion, surgery was the only really viable option.

I remember lying on the bed at this point being somewhat frustrated as our plans changed again, but deep down, I knew his arguments made sense. Shortly after agreeing, I met with a world-renowned heart surgeon at my bedside. We had a thorough conversation, and it became clear that the preferred option really was surgery. Tom (as he introduced himself) specializes in "minimally invasive heart surgery." That sounded like an oxymoron to me; isn't all open-heart surgery pretty invasive? He explained that minimally invasive surgery is surgery that doesn't include cutting through the sternum (breastbone) as traditional heart surgery does. The incision is typically under the right breast for a woman;

therefore, visible scarring is minimal. The technique may or may not involve the use of robots to assist. During my surgery, however, they determined that using robots wasn't possible, given the complexity and positioning of my defects.

As I look at my scar today, I am still in wonderment as to how this gifted surgeon was able to angle his instruments through my ribcage without breaking any bones all within a six-inch incision. People travel from around the world to have Tom as their surgeon, and I practically stumbled upon him. I consider myself very fortunate in many ways.

The doctors all left the bedside after Tom explained the procedure, leaving Don and me to decide our course of action. I was fearful at this point and somewhat confused, but the medical advice was now clear. I phoned my brother in the UK and talked through the decision with him and informed him that we were trying to schedule the surgery for that same week although we had been informed that this would be difficult to achieve. We cancelled the percutaneous procedure and then attempted to schedule surgery for three days later. Although this was near impossible, the nurses and assistants were able to pull this off; the tentative date for the surgery was Friday, March 26, just three days away. That afternoon, we began the scheduling and the planning. Scheduling heart surgery is no easy task with just a three-day lead-in, and whilst I was scared at how quickly this was moving, I was very grateful that we didn't have to return to Vegas and wait weeks before coming back to Cleveland in another month.

I had done a relatively reasonable job of holding back my tears until the reality of the situation began to sink in. My tears were of fear when I knew that open-heart surgery was the only real option. To all the doctors and nurses at the clinic, my findings and decision were a major success and an extremely fortunate turn of events, but I was still dealing with the fear.

The three days between the procedures went by fast. One of the people I called was my swim coach. My coach is a very practical man and keeps his emotions to himself mostly, but our conversation was a difficult one. I believe he gets almost as much pleasure coaching me to success as I do achieving it. He has pushed me beyond my limits and has wanted nothing more than to get the best of me through planned and intense training. He wanted me to achieve my Ironman dream. I could tell he was concerned, but true to his form, he kept his emotions to himself and instead talked about when we would resume training. Training for an Ironman is a serious commitment. My program typically involves more than 20 hours per week of training, in some combination of swimming, biking, and running. Add to that a few more hours of strength training and stretching, and it's easy to see how this must become a lifestyle to be achievable. Usually, I train twice a day, once in the morning at 5:30 a.m. and the other in the evening around 6:30 p.m., varying intensities, burning and consuming many calories. I like the discipline of this long-distance endurance event. I had completed in five half Ironman events, each one delivering a sense of accomplishment so overpowering it was enough to get me through any future training blues, which of course were inevitable. I've dreamed of crossing that Ironman finish line, receiving the medal and tee shirt, and getting the obligatory M-dot tattoo, joining a small, elite group of the population.

The evening before the surgery, two close friends of mine from Bermuda called me. While I was pleased to hear their voices and words of encouragement, the conversations were very emotional as they too struggled to understand the situation and deal with its gravity. I also spoke with my brother later that night and insisted at the start of the conversation that we both remain positive, as now it was important for me to get into a positive state of mind. No more tears. No more fear. As I lay awake in the hotel bed that night before the surgery, my brain began to rationalize everything. This was no longer a choice; my surgeon was one of the best in the world, as was this hospital, and he had promised me that my heart would restart. I was becoming more positive, and my brain was getting on board with the concept. It is amazing how powerful rationalization is and how something that was so incomprehensible a few days before can seem like a logical option just a few days later.

On Friday March 26, the morning of my surgery, I awoke early after catching only a few hours of sleep. (I've begun to realize the human body can function pretty well on just a few sleep hours per night; that's all I had for the first few months of 2010.) The pre-op nurse had instructed me that I had to shower using a strong antibacterial soap wash, which she had given to me during our briefing the previous day, once the night before and once the morning of the surgery. In addition to this, I had to apply a nasal antibacterial gel three times: twice the night before and once the morning of the surgery.

Preparing for surgery takes time, and I had only had three days to get there physically and mentally. More blood had been drawn and another chest X-ray done, as well as yet another ultrasound, this time of my groin, to ensure that the flow of blood in my femoral arteries was normal. The ultrasound was performed at 7:00 a.m. on Thursday 25 March in the vascular medicine center by a technician who clearly hadn't had sufficient caffeine by that time in the morning. I also met with an anesthesiologist that same day and gave him the details of my not-so-great reaction to the general anesthetic following my knee surgery. The evening following my knee surgery, I had felt very nauseated. This hadn't subsided until after I had filled a plastic bag full of saline vomit. Anesthesia and I don't go well together. Apparently, the smaller and fitter you are, the more it can affect you. I was about to find out (a few days later) that my intolerance for medication still existed despite the anti-nausea meds.

I also was scheduled for a latex allergy test, and even though the result was negative, there was an adhesive intolerance that concerned the surgical team such that they ordered a complete set of latex-free material and equipment for my surgery.

We had been instructed to arrive at 10:30 the morning of the surgery to the admitting desk and family waiting area. I was immediately escorted back to a preparation ward and instructed to undress and, for the second time that week, put on the hospital gown. My vital signs and weight were taken, and again, I was instructed to provide a urine sample to ensure I wasn't pregnant. My word was, of course, still not proof enough for this, and neither was the negative result from the test three days prior! Like all surgical patients, I had been told that eating and drinking anything after midnight was forbidden. Having been scheduled for an afternoon operation, I felt this was unfair, as I was already feeling dehydrated despite the fact that I had purposely drunk bottle after bottle of water until 11:59 p.m. in an attempt to prevent dehydration. When I questioned this logic to a nurse, she simply explained that if a morning procedure was cancelled for some reason, the afternoon procedure would be brought forward and therefore the patient would need to have avoided food and fluid since midnight. This seemed logical.

Don was paged and allowed to come back to the preparation ward and to my cubicle. We sat, chatted, and waited for two and a half hours for the call. I read magazines and books and e-mailed and texted with friends, but it was one of the longest waits of my life. The nurses were reassuring and checked in with me regularly to tell me there was no change and that the anticipated time for my procedure was still 1:30 p.m. My emotions were hard to keep under control during this time. I was beyond turning back, and the only way through this was to continue to focus on the positives and the statistics. I fought hard not to give in to the ever-present thoughts of fear and death. Looking back, I'm not sure I really know how I got through that morning mentally; like in most stressful situations, the body and mind can act in miraculous ways, and perhaps my mind went into a sort of autopilot mode and I just somehow got through it.

I was interviewed by the nurse and asked what my anxiety level was on a scale of 1 to 10. I replied it was a 10 and then asked her if anyone waiting for heart surgery ever had an answer that was less than 10. She claimed that the person she asked before me had replied with a 2 because he saw his surgery as the only option for him to live a healthy life. About an hour before I was finally called, I had a visit from one of the hospital chaplains. Looking back, I understand this is an important part for some patients, because they talk and pray together, but I felt in some strange way that by praying with the chaplain, I was a little closer to accepting death as a possibility. I wasn't mentally ready to go there and was trying desperately not to, so although I longed to chat and pray with her, I declined and thanked her. Instead, I privately reached out to God as I do each and every night and trusted I was in good hands.

Finally, around 1:30 p.m., the nurses came to transport me to the pre-op room. In the movies, your loved ones surround your bed as you are wheeled to the operating room, and your loved ones tell you that they love you and you should be strong. Hands are held and lasting kisses given. I was determined not to cry during this moment, and when the nurse finally told Don this was as far as he could go, I was secretly praying that he would not tell me he loved me, as I already knew that and the words would cause tears, which would achieve nothing, only adding to my stuffed-up nose. I smiled at Don and told him I would see him in a few hours. He said it was just like doing an Ironman, and he therefore wished me good luck and said he would see me at the finish line. Perfect. I held it together and soon was in the pre-op room, with much activity happening around me.

First things first: I explained again (for the third time that week) that I was recovering from a cold, my nose was blocked, and I had the remnants of a sore throat. All the literature that I had read mentioned that having a cold may result in a postponement of surgery. None of the nurses were concerned; they checked my temperature and explained that unless I was suffering from a fever and was perhaps 30 years older, the surgery would be going ahead. I'm not sure if I was secretly hoping that it wouldn't at that point. Who knows?

The nurses began the tasks of inserting three IVs. This took considerably longer than normal, as I am officially classed as a tough stick. This means that finding easily accessible veins in my arms and hands to insert IVs into is a tough task for the nurses. This had been a constant problem over the past few weeks at the clinic. One of the IVs the nurses were inserting was to hook me up to a saline drip, one was for my general anesthesia meds, and one, the largest needle, was to directly and more accurately monitor my heart rate, oxygen levels, and blood pressure. After two failed attempts, (which later resulted in a five-inch bruise on my arm) all needles were finally "in." I met with two of the anesthesiology team in the pre-op room; the doctor in charge was less than cheery and did not even try to sugarcoat the fact that in all likelihood, I would have a negative reaction to the general anesthetic. Not great.

Then it was time. My legs were strapped down and my head positioned on a small hollow sponge "pillow." The nurses wheeled me into my operating room. The room was cold and teeming with people busy doing tasks. I was hooked up to all the IVs and machines. Within minutes, I felt tired. One of the anesthetists told me he would make me comfortable and I would feel tired and could go to sleep if I wanted while they ran through their pre-op routines. They would wake me when Tom arrived and he would then run through the plan. I was tired and slipped into an instant sleep. I suspect I was given valium or one of its relatives, but I'm not sure.

I was awakened by Tom gently saying my name close to my face and touching my shoulder. I have no idea how long I was asleep for. Tom was smiling as I opened my eyes; I asked him if it was over, and he smiled again, saying it hadn't yet begun. I remember him addressing his medical team with his surgical plan. I wish I could remember what he said, but all I remember is him looking at me and asking if I agreed with the plan. I smiled and said it sounded good to me. That was the last thing I remember.

I asked Don to fill in the gaps…

Before saying good-bye, I told Elle this was just like doing an Ironman. I said good luck and "I'll see you at the finish line."

I went back to the family waiting room for about an hour. The whole day had been very clearly mapped out for family members; all we didn't know was exactly what time Elle would go in for her surgery. I already had a pager that would work anywhere on campus. They would page me with that when it was time to get the families together for a briefing and then when Elle's surgeon came out of surgery to give me an update. In the meantime, it was one long waiting game. There were all types of people in the waiting room, young and old, different backgrounds and ethnicities, but all had the same sort of look on their faces—sort of a glassy-eyed look, a little like everything happening was a bit surreal. Everyone had different approaches to keeping busy—some were read-ing, some chatting, some playing games and cards, some watching television, some obsessing over their iPhones. After reading for a little while, I found a quiet corner to open my laptop. I'd been away from work for a while and it had not been expected, so I was continually trying to keep up with what was happening back at the hotel and keep the e-mails up to date. It was a good way to occupy my mind.

I spoke to the ladies at the desk and let them know I was going to take a walk. I paid the obligatory visit to Starbucks, of course, and then headed back to the hotel for a change of clothes and a quick walk outside for some fresh air. Then I headed back to the waiting room, as my pager had gone off—it was only about 3:00 p.m. which seemed far too quick to hear about the surgery—I hoped that everything was going okay but couldn't help but think something might be wrong. Thankfully, though, everything was fine; all the families were being called to a briefing session by one of the senior nurses on what to expect after surgery and all the dos and don'ts.

A couple of days earlier, Elle and I had watched a video showing us what to expect after surgery in the ICU. It was certainly a very ethereal experience and made everything seem very real. Elle got completely rattled at this point and was really uncertain that we were doing the right thing, having the surgery. I knew it was and stayed calm, reassuring her that we really had to do this—I couldn't imagine the consequences of doing nothing. Fortunately, Tom, Elle's surgeon, echoed my thoughts, explaining that this was not a counseling session after which we had a choice to make—this was no longer elective, it was a necessity. His very calm but clear demeanor really helped us through this very difficult time.

Nonetheless, however hard it was to watch that video, it set the stage in my mind for what to expect, and it would certainly have been much worse to walk into the ICU with no realization of what I would be facing.

The nurse explained again what it would be like in the ICU. We were warned that depending on how the surgeries went, we might not get in until about 8:00 p.m. and we would only be allowed in for 20-30 minutes so the patients would not get overburdened and so the nurses could take best care of them.

We were reminded to stay close and to keep the pagers with us, as the surgeon would come and talk to us after the surgery was complete and that would be any time from 5:00 p.m. onwards. We were told where the ICU was and that we should report there about two hours after we met with the surgeon.

I was given good advice on things to say to Elle, such as "I know you can't talk to me," "You have done so well, and you look really good," and a rather alarming "Your hands are restrained so that you don't pull out the breathing tube"! We were reminded that our phones should be off in the ICU (a perfectly good reason not to take any calls from work, I thought) and then were told specifics about our loved ones.

"Ellen Charnley—started on the heart at 2:39 p.m. You need to report to ICU at J5."

One by one, families shuffled out and back to the waiting room. I spoke to a couple of people back at work after that, which seemed like a good idea to keep my mind busy, and then during one call, my pager went off and I had to remind myself to say something rather than just hang up and run to the desk.

I was told that the surgeon was on his way down to meet me—it all seemed to happen so quickly. I can't remember the exact time this happened, but it seemed like it was far too soon—he had either worked really quickly or maybe something had not gone well. I knew this was not that case as soon as I saw Tom—he was smiling and very quickly told me that the operation had been a complete success. He had been able to use the minimally invasive technique as planned (so did not have to go through the sternum) although without the help of robotics. He had completely replaced the wall of Ellen's heart. He said that the wall of the heart had been in a much worse condition than we had expected, describing it as a piece of "wet tissue paper," which didn't sound too good. He also confirmed that this surgery was the only course of action that would have kept her alive; they would not have been able to repair the wall using the occluders, as there were too many holes in her heart and they were spread far across the whole wall, and not least because the wall was too flimsy to allow anything to be attached to it. He explained that he had taken some of her pericardium (the sack that the heart sits in) and built an entirely new wall. Once the wall was repaired, he had noticed that with the blood flowing correctly in the heart, the side of her heart that had grown disproportionate in size had already started reducing in size.

So, all was well and we now just had to focus on her recovery—he thought she would be up and running in no time!

He headed off, and I sat there for a few moments taking everything in and adjusting my mental approach. With the relief that came with the news I knew that all the uncertainties were now to be removed from my mind and I had to get into full confidence mode and prepare to support Elle through recovery.

I handed in my pager and went back to the hotel for an hour or so. After I sent out a few quick e-mail updates, I then went over to the new waiting room at J5, where I was given another pager. This time I sat reading until finally I was called to go through. I braced myself, remembering the images and descriptions and getting ready to go into full positivity mode.

I turned around the corner, and Elle was there just like in the video, with pipes, tubes and IVs everywhere—she was awake although a little *delirious and obviously not comfortable. The nurse did a lot of talking, giving me all sorts of updates of what had happened since Elle arrived and what the monitors were telling us. Some of this explanation was done in a quieter voice so that Elle could not hear her. The breathing tube would likely remain in for a few more hours. All Elle wanted to know was when it would come out. As we communicated, we knew that she could not see a clock, and so the answer to this question was always vague: "in a little while" or "maybe another hour." The nurse explained that because Elle was young and fit, likely she wouldn't have to keep it in for too long but there is nothing worse than taking it out too soon and having to put it back in.*

Communication becomes a full-time job when you can't speak. The nurse had been trying to answer questions that Elle had been writing out on the palm of her hand. So I started this little game with Elle—it's very hard, especially when your game partner is dozing on and off. We started with initials of words and then tried to guess the rest. We answered most of the questions—the most common one being, How much longer for the tube, the second most common one being, What is the beeping, is my heart stopping? All night she was really worried about her heart rate dropping. The monitor was set to send an audible alarm if Elle's heart rate dropped below a certain limit just for safety. Unfortunately, every time Elle heard it, she must have thought her heart was stopping. She needed to rest, but every time she dozed off, her heart slowed down, the monitor went off again, and she panicked.

The guessing game seemed to be getting harder, so we graduated to pen and paper. (Why didn't we think of that earlier?) Well, to my surprise, I was quickly ready to revert to the writing on the palm of my hand. I kept the envelope with Elle's scribbles on it so she could see why I wasn't able to answer her every question instantly. Those are the scribbles on the front of this book.

The nurse was fantastic—so calm and reassuring—and I just joined her in constantly telling Elle how well she was doing and everything I knew from the day. I told her how well the surgery had gone and how pleased Tom was and also how many people had been in contact, asking how she was. We held hands a lot, and I plugged in her iPod to her favorite David Gray album, which really helped to keep her calm.

Finally, the hour came when they were ready to remove the dreaded breathing tube. A male nurse came round and went through a series of checks and tests and then told Elle everything to do and to expect. He was one of many who were very chatty when he realized we lived in Vegas and was very excited to tell me that he would be there next month—everyone seems to have a reason to come to Vegas at some point. I don't think Elle was terribly interested in his travel plans, though, and finally, he removed her breathing tube and she took her first step toward recovery.

Her voice was weak, raspy, and higher than usual, but it was great to hear her speaking. I could sense such a difference that this first hurdle was over, we both felt so much better.

Before I knew it, it was after midnight. The nurse told me that it was time for me to head out, as Elle needed to rest. I slowly realized how tired and hungry I was—I had expected to get kicked out by 9:00 p.m. and hadn't eaten. I had been allowed to stay much longer than the anticipated 20-30 minutes.

I gave Elle a kiss good night and told her everything was going brilliantly and that I'd be back in the morning. I thanked the nurse—how lucky we were to have her looking after Elle all night, everyone was fantastic.

I headed out into the hospital, suddenly starving, only to find that almost everything was closed. I managed to find a pot of macaroni and cheese and took it back to the hotel, were I finished it off while sending out all sorts of great news messages to people to let them know how well Elle was doing. It was 2:00 a.m. before I got into bed, and I lay there for a while thinking about how lucky we were to be there and in such great hands.

The nurses in the cardiac wards work 12-hour shifts. During this time, they check on their patients typically five or six times. They give medication, either by capsule or IV, draw blood and ask how the patients are feeling, talk about progress and next steps (which tube they will remove next!), and so on. In addition to the nurses, there is a team of nursing assistants; I presume they work 12-hour shifts also, but I never asked that question. The nursing assistants take vital signs every four hours without fail and help the nurses with the less medical aspects of caring for the patients, such as bathing and physically assisting them with movement. They check four vital signs: body temperature, blood pressure, heart rate, and oxygen level. Body temperature is taken with a traditional thermometer placed under the tongue, blood pressure and heart rate with a blood pressure cuff, and oxygen level with a small matchbox-like device placed over the tip of the forefinger. Normal readings for me for these vital signs are (1) 96–97 degrees, (2) 95–100 over 50–60, (3) 45–55 beats per minute (bpm), and (4) 97–100%. During my stay in hospital, my vital signs are generally within these ranges, but there are some instances when my heart rate and blood pressure drop significantly, and at one point, my oxygen levels fall during sleep, at which point I have to be placed back on the oxygen pipes that gently provide oxygen into my nostrils.

Blood clots are a concern for most postoperative patients, so to help prevent these, electronic massaging stockings are placed around the calves to gently and consistently massage the calves and move blood through the legs. I find this relaxing and somewhat enjoyable, but the machine the stockings are hooked up to is located at the end of my bed and next to Don's head whilst he tries to sleep, so he is finding it less enjoyable.

It is now Saturday evening, and the nausea is more intense. I also have an intense headache. I reach for a bowl and rest my head slightly above it should I vomit. I'm attached to an automatic pain medication pump; I can press it to release more, and this not only reduces my pain as I cough and move but also makes me drowsy. I drift in and out of consciousness, and the drugs get me through the night. Don leaves for an hour to take a shower in the hotel room, and he speaks with Emily, my night nurse, and asks her to stay in the room with me for an hour until he returns. I am happy Emily is with me, as my pain and anxiety are returning and there are new pains in my back that I am unfamiliar with. Emily sits at the end of my bed and "charts" silently. I am grateful to Emily. Don returns, and Emily tends to her other patients. Don sleeps on the couch at the end of my bed. I am happy he is with me. I don't really notice Emily returning into my room that night to check my vital signs and change my IV bag. She opens my mouth and inserts the thermometer and reaches for my arm, then slips out of the room quietly in the dark. I'm not aware of very much that night; I drift in and out of consciousness as Don sleeps on and off.

Sunday morning, March 28, I still feel nauseated, but I think eating something may help; that's what everyone is trying to convince me to do anyway. The breakfast tray arrives and consists of a very unappetizing omelet, some juice, and some bran flakes. I attempt a few mouthfuls of the flakes but within the hour regret it. Finally, I vomit into the closely positioned bowl. I feel significantly better. Linda is back on duty to take care of me. She gives me more pain meds and more antinausea medicine. I am exhausted and sleep for a couple of hours in the afternoon. As I awake, Linda is in my room and checking my vital signs. She is so cheery; the sun shines through the window. Linda seems happy to tell me that I look better and that Don took a walk to get some fresh air. Linda suggests we try to move from the bed to the chair. What an adventure. I agree, and Linda places a waterproof sheet on the chair. The move takes at least five minutes to achieve. The effort tires me. My nausea has temporarily subsided.

Sitting in a chair is one step closer to recovery. The next step, Linda explains, is to remove the urinary catheter. This would mean I could then wear underwear and a sanitary napkin and take some element of control of my bodily functions back, slightly less humbling than lying on a waterproof sheet. Linda positions herself on the floor in front of me and explains how she will deflate the balloon that is holding the catheter in place. She does this and gently pulls on the tube until it releases painlessly. One more tube removed. One more step to recovery.

I eat some crackers and more ice chips. Don returns and we watch a movie together. My nausea and headache return. I am mentally exhausted from this feeling; the two days already seem too many. That second night in J5-3 is a long one. I awake frequently, coughing regularly, and my back pain is increasing.

The nurses typically deal with most routine medical issues themselves, but if they need to order meds or tests, then they consult with the doctor on call for the ward. That night, the doctor comes to visit me and orders a mobile chest X-ray as a result of my persistent coughing. The portable X-ray machine is brought to my bed, and a metal plate is placed behind my back while two nurses lift me into position. The movement causes an increase in my pain. The X-ray will reveal whether I have started to accumulate fluid on my lungs, another concern with open-heart surgery patients who have been placed on heart-lung machines. The X-ray is normal in that regard. A few drugs are administered to me that night, and, finally, a combination of lidocaine patches, new meds, and a back massage from Nurse Joe help me to get more comfortable by 5:00 a.m. Joe is a senior male nurse in the cardiac ward, and his experience caring for post–heart-surgery patients is clearly evident. His ability to massage my back at just the right intensity and location is amazing; his hands feel magical, and my backache subsides.

The nausea continues through Monday morning, and after another attempt to vomit the remaining few ounces of fluid from my stomach, I finally started to feel better.

Rehabilitation is not the same for every cardiac patient. As an athlete, my expected recovery was supposedly fast, plus, surgery wasn't to correct cardiac disease or thickening arteries due to ill health, smoking, or obesity; I was born with my defects. The instruction to begin walking around the ward is the same for everyone, however. Because of my nausea, I didn't achieve my first sprint around J5-3 with Don until that Monday morning. By Monday afternoon, we attempted an Olympic-distance triathlon—well, two full circuits of the ward. The doctor who visited that morning insisted that we begin walking because this would make me feel better and allow my body to start functioning fully again, and by that, he meant generating a bowel movement.

On Monday afternoon, I leave my room for an hour by wheelchair as transportation takes me to X-ray for another chest X-ray and then to radiology for a post-op echo of my new heart. Both are normal. My echo is truly miraculous to watch on screen. My heart pumps blood only in the direction that it should, and not an ounce of blood passes between the upper chambers. This is confirmation that my new heart is fully functioning and my surgeon has repaired the wall and the holes. As I wait for transportation to come and collect me, I chat to another patient. She looks in pain and looks sick. I wonder what she thinks I look like. She is a heart-surgery patient also but has been in hospital for a full week. She hopes to be discharged today. I feel a sense of warming to this patient, my first real connection with someone going through something similar to myself. We both wish each other a speedy recovery.

By Monday evening, March 29, I only have two IVs left, the central line in my neck and one in my left arm. If you are admitted to hospital it is likely that you will have at least one IV, and you can only be discharged once all the IVs are removed. I eat more crackers and drink more fluid, and this time they stay down. We determine that I am better off without the antinausea medicine. Nurse Mia has been with me all day and is doing a double shift so will be with me until 11:00 p.m. Mia tells me I have to take potassium, as my potassium levels are too low. To reduce my water retention, I had been placed on a diuretic; this had caused my potassium levels to drop. Potassium affects the functioning of the heart, so I have no choice; I have to take the potassium. The only choice Mia gives me is the method, either by IV (which would sting, apparently) or by large horse-like pills, four of them. Now, for someone who has only just started to keep any food or liquid down, I know this will be difficult. Taking meds is a supervised process. The potassium is not optional, and Mia watches me swallow hard. The process takes several minutes before all four tablets leave my mouth. As Mia closes the door behind, the fourth pill returns from my stomach; I don't tell her.

It is Tuesday morning, March 30. The doctor comes into my room on his rounds. He unbuttons my gown and inspects my incisions and my vital signs. He asks about my bowel movement or lack thereof and about how I am feeling. He instructs the nurse to remove the central line and says I should be able to be discharged this afternoon. Normally, having a bowel movement is a prerequisite for being discharged, but I am given a day's reprieve because I've eaten next to nothing;

however, this is only on the proviso that I take a double portion of laxative—supervised, of course.

Jess is my nurse today; she delicately begins to remove the sutures around the central line in my neck. This is painful; without control, tears roll down my cheeks. Jess works fast and apologizes for the pain. Finally, the line is out and I am left with three small holes in my neck. I now am just hooked up to the monitor and have one IV left in my arm.

Today I am allowed to take a shower. The only remaining IV, however, must be covered up completely, with waterproof tape. I am also instructed to use the chair, which is carefully positioned, in the center of the extra-large shower. I am allowed to use only baby shampoo and cannot remain in the shower for long. I scrub at the yellow surgical iodine stain all over my body, but I am unsuccessful in removing it with nothing more than simple soap and water. Nevertheless, the smell of fresh soap is sweetly overpowering and I am thankful that I no longer smell and feel stale. The nursing assistant checks in on me, and I report that I am doing just fine. I ask her if I can wear my own clothes or whether I have to wear another hospital gown. She tells me she'll check with Jess and let me know. I am hanging onto the words the doctor mentioned this morning about being discharged today, although that now seems a long time ago. Jess returns and tells me to get dressed in my own yoga pants and tee shirt. I really am going to be discharged today.

Taking a shower is a long process from start to finish, and I am once again exhausted and retreat back to my bed. Jess removes the waterproof taping, and then we wait for the discharge papers to be collected. This is a long wait. I am not allowed to be an inpatient without being hooked up to the monitors, so even though the expected timeframe before my discharge is less than two hours, Jess places fresh electrode pads over my chest and abdomen again, and the monitor records my heart rhythms. Thankfully, she allows me to stay dressed in my own clothes. At 1:00 p.m., lunch arrives—turkey and gravy. I am finally getting my appetite back; however, just at the same moment, transportation arrives and I am finally discharged and allowed to return to my hotel room for a couple more days. I never get to eat the lunch, but I am relieved; I am one step closer to recovery. I am anxious, though; no more caregivers other than Don to check on me every four hours. What if something should go wrong?

CHAPTER 3

My Hotel Room

March 2010

Don collects my belongings. I am wheeled to the connecting hotel and to our hotel room, which I haven't seen in five days. We watch movies and daytime television, and I begin to call my friends and family, now feeling strong enough mentally and physically to begin to tell my story and reassure everyone that I am on the road to recovery.

The first night outside the hospital is a long one. I am restless, and my anxiety level is high. I finally begin to doze off around 5:00 a.m., but I am almost sitting upright in the bed to alleviate my back and shoulder pain. I sleep until 9:00 a.m., and then Don and I take a 20-yard walk from our hotel room to the club lounge for breakfast. I still have no sense of taste, and my tongue is white, not pink (a common side effect from the general anesthesia), but I am happy to be sitting upright for breakfast in the lounge and chatting to the hotel staff, even if I eat very little. One of the staff members, Antoinette, greets me and is pleased to have me back in the hotel. She treats all the recovering patients as her family, and she is truly a wonderfully warm person to have around.

I still experience the back pain at night, and I become exhausted very quickly, but we are able to extend our walks outdoors around the clinic campus. The weather is surprisingly warm, and our highlight is a walk to the pharmacy to pick up my meds. A journey that would normally take minutes, we make last an hour. Walking for a longer period of time is a challenge in these early days not only because of the exhaustion and the lightheadedness I feel from the medication but also because I am still in significant pain in my groin from the inch-long incisions and subsequent baseball-size hematoma that has now formed. This apparently is normal and will take several weeks to disappear. Try walking with a baseball in your groin; it's a little difficult.

On Wednesday, I have an appointment with a nurse practitioner in the cardiac center of the clinic. She checks my incisions and vital signs and orders another blood draw to check the potassium levels. The results are normal. She gives me her business card and tells me to call her if I have questions later or when I am back in Vegas. She goes through my discharge papers and my medications and instructs me to make an appointment with my primary care physician within a week.

On Thursday, I meet with a cardiologist, who repeats much of the same but also spends time explaining what will happen as my body heals, the additional pain I will likely feel as the nerve endings grow back in my breast. He candidly explains that although a cut to the sternum (as in traditional open-heart surgery) takes longer to heal, it is reportedly less painful than the quicker-to-heal minimally invasive surgery. Now they tell me!

Each day, I shower and scrub more of the yellow paint away. My neck is still showing the incisions and looks as if I have been stabbed. Other hotel guests stare at me in the hotel lounge and most likely wonder what my story is. The hotel staff do not stare because ill-looking patients are common place in the hotel.

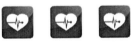

As a child, I was a jack of all trades and master of none, or so my father told me on numerous occasions. If there was one thing I did fairly consistently and competitively between the ages of 7 and 14, however, it was swimming. And I swam quite well—that is, until I grew tired of going to practice and chose other, more appealing pastimes for a teenager. Nevertheless, those seven years of swimming competitively and consistently were enough to provide a great springboard for me compared with the average newbie triathlete. My teenage years and early twenties were somewhat athletically inactive, and it wasn't until I was 24 that I understood the importance of regular exercise and started running and competing in local half-marathon events that Don was racing in. I was only ever averagely talented at pure running, however.

Don and I left the UK in 1996 and have had the privilege of working and living in some extremely desirable places: Bermuda, San Francisco, Hawaii, and now Las Vegas. It was in Bermuda that I became more passionate about fitness and soon began a second career alongside accountancy and became a certified personal fitness trainer and spinning instructor. This became my only focus in San Francisco, and there, I first started thinking about the sport of triathlon; however, the closest I came to ever taking up the sport was to purchase a road bike. Our time in San Francisco came to an abrupt end when Don was transferred to Hawaii, and it was in Hawaii that I joined a local non-elite triathlon club called Team Jet. Here my passion was born, and I have been a triathlete ever since. I competed locally in the short- and medium-length races, termed "sprint" and "Olympic" distances and generally placed high in my age group. I was still relatively young, so injuries were not yet plaguing me.

Eventually, I became interested in training and racing in longer-distance events and finally signed up for a half Ironman distance event called Eagleman in Baltimore. At the time, this was one of the hardest events I had ever completed. I wanted to quit many times during the half marathon leg, but I endured and crossed the finish line, and my passion for longer distance events was born. I experienced a sense of accomplishment I had never experienced before, and it is this sense that keeps me driven to achieve more. I did reasonably well in that event and ended up qualifying for the world age-group championships in Florida a few months later. I continued to race this distance each year as my main focus. Finally, in 2009, I believed I was ready for the big one, double this distance, the full Ironman, and in November 2009, I signed up for the 2010 Ironman Arizona. Signing up for an

Ironman is a difficult task. Oddly, this grueling event is increasing in popularity, and today, you need to sign up a year in advance for most races, and they sell out within minutes.

On Friday, April 2, just one week after my surgery, we are flying home to Las Vegas. I have mixed feelings as we pack our bags and gather my voluminous medical records. We have been fortunate enough to meet with Linda from the clinic's executive services team. Through some business associates of Don's, word had reached the clinic that we were to be taken care of; this we found quite humbling, but we appreciated the care and attention that Linda gave us those two weeks. Linda had helped with scheduling the surgery, visited me in the hospital, and also gathered up my file of medical records for me to take home. We are truly grateful for the help that Linda gave us.

I am almost sad to be leaving the place that has been my home and safe place for two weeks, but I am also happy to be homeward bound, one more step closer to recovery. I am also excited to see our little dog, Dude, who has been in my positive thoughts and imagery these past weeks. I am apprehensive, though; walking my dog will be tough for a few days, and he will no doubt be frustrated with me for my slow pace. April will be my refocus and rebalance month and my appreciate-every-thing-that-life-has-to-offer month. At the end of April, I will reassess my Ironman goals and consider if they are indeed realistic for November 2010.

My family—Mum, Dad, and my brother and his family—all still live in the UK. Because of the speed of actions and decisions that we made, telling my parents was something I had chosen not to do. My mum was always the one who would make everything better when I was a little girl, but she would not have been able to wave her magic wand this time from afar, nor would she have been able to get to Cleveland in time. Telling her would not have achieved very much and would have made her life temporarily miserable with worry, resulting in an additional burden to me also. I did, however, get comfort from discussing every-thing with my brother. Paul and I were very close as kids, but geo-graphically, we are separated, which adds limitations to our contact; however, something has remained strong between us, and he was a pil-lar of strength during my days at the clinic. He supported my decision not to burden my parents.

CHAPTER 4

Stages of Grief

I had heard about the stages of grief many years ago during a work-sponsored seminar I attended. I don't believe I spent too long thinking about these at the time, and, fortunately, I have not had cause to during my life—that is, until this year. I researched the stages on the Internet, as I was certain that I had subconsciously experienced these all during a short space of time at the hospital.

Denial: I know I felt fine. I didn't believe there was anything wrong with me, even when I was shown that first echo image on the screen in the doctor's office, I thought, *So what, I have a few holes in my heart? Well if I've had them all my life, then who cares? Let me get on with my life and, more importantly, with my training.*

Anger: Why me? It's not fair. Once in the second stage, the individual recognizes that denial cannot continue. I know this stage occurred, as more and more medical professionals reiterated my condition and the seriousness of it. I became frustrated that I was one of the 1% of the population who was born with a defect.

Bargaining: Just before I went into surgery, my emotions ran wild, and there is no question that I tried to subconsciously bargain with God. As the reality slipped into my mind that there was a chance that I may not wake up, I began thinking of all the things that I would promise to do if I woke up. This third stage involves the hope that the individual can somehow postpone or delay the negative outcome.

Depression: It was very hard leaving the familiar and safe surroundings of the hospital and returning to Vegas to begin my recovery, not being able to swim, ride, or run, and becoming easily exhausted from walking my dog. Depression is very common for heart-surgery patients. There is much research done on the heart-lung machine and how it affects the brain post surgery, creating a depressed state. The severity of my condition and the significance of these events humbled me, scared me, and ultimately depressed me for several weeks.

Acceptance: When my surgeon assertively told me that I had no choice about the surgery and that my heart would fail, a switch occurred in my brain; I began to accept my fate, to accept what God had in store for me, and to simply deal with it. I felt a sense of peace because I was no longer fighting the diagnosis or the question of surgery. This was now decided, and what would be would be.

Did I ever think of dying? Did I imagine my heart stopping? Yes. Death is something all heart-surgery patients think of at some point, of that I am certain—some, I suspect, more than others. I did think of death, and I did worry about my heart failing, particularly in those early days post surgery. In the ICU, my fear was fear of death, but, quite unexplainably, the fear was rationally accepted by my brain. I certainly did not wish to die, but for a few brief moments, I think I understood that the fear was unnecessary and that God would decide my fate; whatever the outcome, I knew that I would be okay. I have often wondered since if this is how terminally ill patients view death when faced with the inevitable. The state of acceptance is not so hard to achieve, and I think for the patient, this state is quicker to achieve than for their loved ones. I doubt that Don ever feared that death was a possibility, but I have never asked him.

CHAPTER 5

Spring in Vegas

April 2010

It's springtime in Vegas, and I look out of our bedroom window. The sun is shining as the trees are gently flowing in the light breeze. It feels good to be home, and I am looking forward to spending time with friends and my dog, who hasn't left my side since we returned home yesterday. I think about how long it will be before I will feel like riding my bike, running the trails, or swimming in Lake Mead. This seems a long way away. But I am one step closer to recovery. Today I plan to take Dude for a long walk, just eight days post surgery. Each day, I am able to do more and more, and I am hoping the recovery period is fast.

 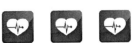

I've never been a particularly fast competitor, and I think this is why I gravitated toward longer distance events; I can normally simply keep going and going. Some sports gurus attribute this to a greater percentage of slow-twitch muscle fibers or endurance fibers rather than fast-twitch fibers. My doctors and, to some extent, I are eagerly waiting with interest to see if my newly fixed heart will provide me with some additional aerobic capacity and athletic improvement. As I sip my morning coffee, I wonder. I know Don is telling everyone I am now "bionic" and will soon be winning races.

I think the general population is somewhat uniformed about heart surgery and, in particular, the medical advancements that have escalated in recent years. Most people hear the words "open-heart surgery" and fear the worst, possibly even a death sentence. I did too, to some extent in the beginning, but the more I learned about open-heart surgery and became somewhat educated, the less I feared it. The mortality rate from the type of surgery that I had is 1%. I heard this statistic from my surgeon, and although this is a low number, it is still 1 in 100. I still think of this, and I wonder when I will no longer. Hospital doctors are faced with a conundrum, telling and educating patients with all the facts and figures but still making sure they stay positive. I had begun to understand the difficulty of this as we spoke to various nurses and doctors. On more than one occasion, I was asked if I had a will and whether my emergency contact was my husband. The Internet is a very powerful tool of modern society. If you type in "open-heart surgery," there are simply thousands of articles that pop up, most of which would scare the reader into an anxiety attack. I am grateful that I didn't have the time to spend hours researching on the Internet before my surgery.

The Adult Congenital Heart Association (ACHA) is a registered charity, supporting awareness for adult congenital heart disorders. Like most people, I wasn't even aware that this charity existed pre surgery; of course, I've now become a member and will look forward to supporting this charity in years to come. I've never been part of a small statistic before, never thought I would be one of those rare percentages. I had always felt that illness or serious conditions happened to others but not me.

My family history is relatively unremarkable; most folk have lived long lives, and there is no recorded evidence of heart disease or congenital defects, cancer or other serious conditions. My maternal grandmother did, however, die from a stroke at the age of 79. I have recently wondered if she had a heart condition. Congenital heart defects are not hereditary; however, the statistics show that if a parent has a

congenital heart defect, there is a 3% (versus a 1% chance)
that a child could have a defect too.

April 16, exactly three weeks post surgery; this week has been a
rough week. Week 2 progressed pretty well, although I was suffering
from periods of vision loss, the kind of vision loss associated with
migraines. These episodes would occur two or three times per day
and leave me useless and confined to the couch for 20 minutes at a
time. There was no pattern or warning. These episodes eventually
subsided. Week three brought more chest and back pain. This was
a new pain that led me back to my primary physician. She did a thorough work-over and sent me for a chest X-ray and EKG. These
results were relatively unremarkable, and she concluded this was all
part of the recovery process and inflammation of the pericardium
(the lining of the heart sac).

I finally set up my bike on my indoor trainer. My plan is to spin my legs
without much effort for approximately thirty minutes. This will be a
stable structure and provide little motion to my upper body; given that
any jolt causes pain in my right breast; I figure this is a good option.
The spinning goes well, but my heart rate monitor proves that the past
few weeks of inactivity have crushed my fitness level. My previous
readings pre-surgery were approximately 135–145 bpm for such an easy
spin. Now my heart is between 150 and 160 bpm. I am concerned this
is too much for my heart to handle, so I ease off. My surgeon had told
me at the clinic that my heart was fixed and that I shouldn't worry about
limiting my exercise. I am still skeptical. Still, this is my first day of real
exercise; my expectations are low.

I progress on my trainer the following week, gradually increasing the
duration to 45 minutes. My heart rate still increases much faster than
before, but I have a lot of fitness to gain. By the weekend, I feel ready
to take my bike outside. Don is keen to come too, mainly to chaperone
me. We take an easy route from our house south to avoid the hilly terrain of Red Rock Canyon, my typical bike route. It feels so wonderful
to be outside, moving and spinning my legs. The air seems fresher than

I remember, and the smells of spring are everywhere. We amble along, barely breaking a sweat, but it still feels good. We stop several times to rest, take in the view, and buy Don's emergency snacks.

Week 5 is done, and not a week I want to repeat anytime soon. I seem to have good weeks followed by bad weeks. Now I am lying on a massage table, my heart is pounding; it is the first time I have lain face down for more than five weeks. It feels strange; my right breast is slightly tender in this position, but that is nothing to the pounding of my heart. Perhaps being in this position is not great for my heart. I can't think why and try hard to reduce any anxiety that is likely causing this. During my triathlon training, I made a point of scheduling regular massages in an attempt to coax my legs and back into thinking they could continue with the heavy demands of my training. At age 41, my body takes longer to recover after workouts. Massage is one of my favorite pastimes, although normally I wince and squirm throughout, as I insist on deep tissue, so it is almost an unbearable experience. Today, I am anxiously waiting for my massage therapist to reenter the room and begin what I hope will be a more gentle massage, my hope being to relax and work out some of the tension in my shoulders and back that has been developing over the past weeks from having to sleep almost upright for many nights. Yesterday, I entered a 5k charity event. Normally, I run these, but yesterday, I had to be happy with a walk. It was an event to raise awareness and funds for breast cancer. I was happy to participate.

This past week, I had two more hospital tests, two more physician visits, and lots of pain. The most frustrating thing was that this was week 5. Shouldn't the pain be reducing, not increasing? Last weekend, I rode my bike outside, for the second time; it was a glorious spring day in Vegas and I was delighted to feel strong enough to take my bike outside. I rode into the mountains, and the sight of Red Rock seemed even more vibrant than before. I was monitoring my heart rate to make sure it didn't climb too high, hard to do when the first 10 miles are a modest incline into the mountains. I felt great and finally experienced the endorphins I'd missed for five weeks when they returned with an added kick that made my day seem simply wonderful. This was what life was about. When I had returned from the ride, I had felt it time to try a stretch and splash in the local lap pool. Moving my arms and attempting swimming was a scary thought. Would my right chest feel more pain? Would I even remember how to pull through a stroke? My first few strokes were hesitant, but I soon increased my momentum and reached a little farther and pulled a little harder with each one. I was swimming again, slowly but very surely. Swimming is like riding a bike in that once you learn your stroke technique, it never really goes away. My chest felt tight, but the swim was good.

Several hours later that night, I had developed chest and back pain. I was relaxing on the sofa when the pain struck and got steadily worse. I figured that I'd pushed my body too hard that morning, so I tried to relax and took some iIbuprofen as instructed by my doctor after the last episode a couple of weeks prior. Each time I took a breath in, I felt a sharp stabbing pain in my back. I tried to relax and to fight the desire to drive to the ER; I figured if the pain didn't get any worse, I could see my doctor in the morning. I didn't sleep that night but sat upright in bed and tried to read a book. The pain was consistent. The following morning, I was able to see my doctor first thing, and she immediately sent me off for further tests, another EKG, of course, and a CT scan of my thoracic region to check for a possible blood clot. Lying flat on my back on the table under the scanner was painful, and I was grateful this wasn't an MRI, which would have taken far longer. The CT scan was with contrast—this means an IV is inserted and at a particular point, iodine dye is injected, which enables the reader of the scan to see a more detailed view. I'd already had a CT scan before, so I knew what to expect when the iodine flowed through my body, but for anyone unfamiliar with this test, let's just say that at an instant a very warm feeling runs through the body and creates the sensation as if you have just peed yourself!

I presumed that since I had not been instantly admitted to the hospital meant no blood clot; however, it wasn't until that evening around 8:30 p.m. that I spoke with my doctor. The pain was increasing, and I was starting to get very concerned, so I called my doctor through her paging system and chatted with her on the phone. She was confident the pain was coming from inflammation of the lining of my heart and possibly my lungs and that the treatment was to take anti-inflammatory medication. There was no clot and nothing different with my EKG. She instructed me to go back on my pain meds that I had received from the Cleveland Clinic, which would, hopefully, allow me to get some sleep. True enough, they knocked me out and I finally slept, albeit upright!

The next day, the pain did start to subside finally, and although not convinced this was the end of it, I was happy taking it one hour at a time. My doctor referred me to a well-regarded local cardiologist, and, given my recent pains, he ordered another echocardiogram of my heart and scheduled an appointment for the next day. His examination of me was pretty thorough, and he was convinced that the pain was inflammation of the lining of the heart, the pericardium, a condition known as pericarditis. This is relatively common in patients following open-heart surgery. He explained to me that my surgery was complex and my body had undergone some major trauma...I knew that, of course, but until that point, I'm not sure I had really, truly understood it. He said this would take some weeks to die down and I shouldn't be alarmed if I experienced further episodes for several more weeks. He, thankfully, was not opposed to me building up my exercise but told me to do so gradually, and he was not of the opinion that exercise had caused this. The method in which the heart-lung machine accesses the heart is through the femoral artery in the groin. The surgeons had made an inch-long incision, which was still healing, and there was significant fluid still causing a large lump. My cardiologist was now concerned about a possible blood clot in that region so ordered an immediate ultrasound.

He called me the following evening to talk about both my echo report and the ultrasound. He explained that the echo showed the repair was intact and that the right side of my heart had started to decrease slightly in size. The ultrasound showed no clot. He was happy with my progress, even if I was slightly frustrated. I realized now that the recovery period of four to eight weeks that surgeons quote really means that will be an approximate period for patients to get to the point where they can work, drive, walk, do groceries, and normal routine activities. This is not the time period that will mean no more pain or that you can run, bike, and swim with any conviction. I was learning the hard way and having to be a patient patient.

I'm recapping this conversation with the cardiologist in my head as I lie on the massage table. My therapist applies pressure to my back, and I start to relax; his hands feel good.

The following week is an up week, with no further complications. I ride my bicycle with a group of friends a couple of times; I even attempt a short swim; whilst that feels rather strange, I am swimming, nonetheless. By the end of the week, I'm considering a short run/walk on the treadmill at the gym. Two days later, I've achieved a 30-minute easy jog. Finally, I start to feel that training for an Ironman maybe possible.

Running and I have never had a perfect relationship. In my mid-twenties, I began running to get fit but had no huge aspirations or ambitions. I had jogged in Wimbledon Common in England and slowly increased my mileage over the years. I learned to enjoy running with music, and now I find races hard with out my iPod in my ear, because most triathlon races ban the use of music or headphones of any kind. I look back now on my running achievements and know, despite periods of consistent and somewhat intense training, I was never ever able to run particularly fast races. My fastest half marathon was 1 hour and 46 minutes on a flat course in California. I wonder now if this was due to cardiovascular limitations.

CHAPTER 6

Back to Work and Training

May 2010

My doctor signs me as fit for work again at the end of April but still keeps a close eye on me and insists I return for weekly visits. I work as a risk management consultant for a large insurance broker, and this involves a fair amount of travel. My first trip of any significance is to visit the Hawaii operation for a week in mid-May. The flight to Hawaii is between six and seven hours, and I have to admit I am a little anxious about making this trip. I am sure to wear my identification bracelet even on the flight. The week is a hectic week full of meetings, and each night, I am exhausted. I continue to exercise to a moderate degree; it's hard not to run along the oceanfront when in Hawaii. This week, I begin to feel some sort of irregular heartbeat, almost as if my heart is skipping a beat. I put it down to anxiety and the additional stress of the work week, but I, of course, discuss this with my cardiologist at my next visit the following week. He sends me for another chest X-ray but is not concerned that this is anything more than just the continuing recovery from the surgery, post-surgical pericarditis. He doubles the anti-inflammatory dose.

During the long flight to and from Hawaii, I began researching other athletes with congenital heart defects. Most notably in the sport of Triathlon is two-time Ironman winner and multiple top-ten finisher professional triathlete Torbjorn Sindballe from Denmark. The well-known, tall Dane is perhaps most remembered for his all-white triathlon race gear in attempt to keep him cool and protect him from the sun and heat. In 2009, Sindballe retired from professional triathlon after being diagnosed with a leaky mitral value, a congenital heart defect. He will at some point require surgery to fix this condition, but for now, he wishes to prolong this requirement and to do this, he has been medically advised to avoid placing his heart in such an exaggerated stress level for prolonged periods of time. When that is your day job, it's time, perhaps, to consider a career change.

As I read about Sindballe, for the first time, I consider that I may be medically advised not to take on the Ironman challenge. I am determined to educate myself as much as possible before I seek medical clearance.

One of my research paths leads me to Dave Watkins. Dave's story is quite extraordinary. He is a fellow triathlete diagnosed with a congenital heart condition and, similar to Sindballe's, his is a valve issue. Dave underwent open-heart surgery in 2005 and suffered significant complications. He has continued to train and race post surgery, but only under the watchful eye of his cardiologist. Dave encourages me to go back to Cleveland for a follow-up meeting with my congenital heart specialist and to seek medical clearance before I embark on any significant training before even contemplating racing in November. Dave has formed a small triathlon team, Ironheart Racing, and I am now a proud member. Ironheart's goal is to raise awareness for the Adult Congenital Heart Association and to raise funds for a number of heart-related charities.

I contact Linda from executive services at the Cleveland Clinic to seek her help in making an appointment back at the clinic. A day later, I receive a call from an assistant at the Cleveland Clinic. She explains that my cardiologist will not give me clearance to race unless he can perform a thorough evaluation and have me undergo some more tests, another echo and a stress echo. We make the appointments and schedule the visit for the end of June. I feel relieved to have a plan and strangely relieved to be going back to Cleveland.

It's Saturday and a holiday weekend. I decide this weekend to ride for a longer period of time, perhaps three hours or more. Before surgery, this duration would have likely caused some blindness in my right eye, so I am curious to see if I will experience this now post surgery. I also would like to report back to the doctors in Cleveland when I return in a few weeks. I ride for 50 miles, which takes me approximately three hours. I ride through Red Rock Canyon, past Blue Diamond, and beyond. The Vegas weather is perfect, not too hot, with no humidity and a light breeze. I continually blink and close my left eye to see if I can see to the same extent out of my right eye. I can. Perhaps the ride isn't long enough to provoke my vision issues, but for now, I'm happy believing that is it and that I am cured.

Riding for longer periods of time gives me time to reflect more and more on the past few weeks. My rides are somewhat emotional for me. During this period, I start to consider if and how I will tell my parents. How would I ever start the conversation? I cannot imagine their reaction, and for now, I still believe that sharing my story with them will provide no benefit, but there is something inside of me that is growing, a sense of betrayal and I start to want to release that burden.

I swim more. I increase my duration and attend my first indoor group swim. Prior to surgery, I would be the fastest swimmer in my triathlon swim group; today, however, I know will be different. I still have a long way to go to build up my cardiovascular fitness. I mentally prepare myself for this fact and take pressure off myself. The session is a success, and I start to feel a little stronger. Next step will be the weekend open-water swim in Lake Mead, my first time in the lake since my Silverman race in November 2009.

I also run. I venture from the safety of the treadmill to the outdoors. I wear my heart rate monitor, of course, and my identification bracelet. I start off slow and steady. Although I feel relaxed and only moderately challenged, my heart rate says otherwise and begins to spike. I slow the pace and walk a little. Prior to surgery, this kind of moderate intensity would have equated to a heart rate of 140–150 bpm. A harder effort would have increased it to 165 but rarely much higher. Now, post surgery, I spike to 176 bpm, yet my perceived exertion is still moderate. This is strange. I take plenty of walk breaks and head home. Eventually, my heart rate settles at a rate of 150 bpm. I make a note of the numbers and discuss with my primary care physician on my next visit. She is still not concerned, but we continue to monitor.

I have a busy month with work. I travel several times to visit clients, and each time, I notice that my heart palpitations increase when I fly. I make a note to discuss this with my cardiologist in Cleveland. Despite the work schedule, I am able to increase my training in all three disciplines quite substantially. My plan is to increase my duration, but not necessarily the intensity so I have a benchmark to discuss with my doctors.

My final weekend of training before heading to Cleveland consists of the following:

> Friday evening—3500-meter swim set
> Saturday morning—4-mile tempo run, followed by 3500-meter lake swim
> Sunday morning—60-mile ride in the desert heat.

CHAPTER 7

Back to Cleveland

June 2010

My heartbeat feels slightly abnormal. It is now a deeper, more exaggerated beat and occasionally seems to skip a beat. I check my pulse, but the count seems normal, around 55 bpm. I've noticed this feeling on a fairly consistent basis each time I fly. I'm thinking about this now, as we fly from Vegas to Cleveland, our third trip this year. I'm listening to ambient sounds on my iPod, coincidentally the same tunes that I listened to over and over again those first few days after my surgery. This trip, I hope, will be different from the last two. Hopefully, there will be no more surprises, no urgent treatment, and, potentially, confirmation that I am healing well and can race Ironman Arizona on November 21.

Don occupies the airline seat next to me and busily types up a report for work on his laptop. For this trip, we decided that it made sense for Don to undergo some general medical testing; with his stressful job (he just opened a hotel in Las Vegas), we believe it's prudent to get him checked out too. Linda, from executive patient services, has arranged a full schedule for Don. In fact, he has more appointments than me this time…well, at least that is the plan, although I'm painfully aware that both previous trips to the clinic have resulted in many more tests and an extended stay each time. I am trying to keep my mind open to this happening again. I am also desperately trying not to get my hopes up; I am half expecting not to receive the green light for racing the Ironman.

I do feel good, though. With the exception of the fluttering heartbeat at times, I have felt continually better through these past few weeks. My training has now increased significantly, and I've started to imagine racing again. I've ridden several four-hour bike rides through the mountains of Red Rock, and all with crystal-clear vision in my right eye. I'm still excited about this finding and hope it continues for future races and long training rides. My running is also progressing well. I'm starting to increase my duration (currently at seven miles) and also some intensity on the shorter runs. My coach has begun to push me on my swim workouts, ever so slightly. I end up breathless at the end of some of sets, and we secretly smile knowingly that if I am given the green light by my doctor, this is the start of a very doable four months of training. He is itching to push me further and harder than last year, but he is wary, I can tell, and so far, he has held back with his workouts and direction.

I have been developing my list of questions over the past month, ever since I scheduled the follow-up visit with my Cleveland cardiologist. They focus on several areas: first, the recovery and the issues I still have regarding the exaggerated heartbeat; training and racing, of course; the possible future complications that I may encounter; and, last, whether there are any hereditary consequences for my family that I may need to inform them about regarding their health. My brother and I have discussed this issue several times over the past month. My research over the past three months has confirmed several relevant points: first that the chances of ASDs being a hereditary condition are were very small and, second, that they are three times more likely in women than in men. Still, I recommended that Paul get an echo, a reliable test to identify any defect, something that the EKG cannot really do. He said he would ask for an appointment, something I thought would be straightforward, until I remembered that the English medical system is more difficult to navigate around and significantly less "urgent" than the US system. He called me back the following week to say he had been referred to a cardiologist, given his "family history" and they would be doing an echo.

This morning, I swam 3500 meters in the pool at my local gym. I can still smell the chlorine on my skin. Smells are such powerful memory-joggers. Chlorine reminds me of my training, of course, but specifically of my childhood swimming for my town club. I think about the smells that are so imprinted on my recent memory, the saline smell and taste in my mouth each time I received an IV, the smell of the sterile yellow iodine painted over my body during the surgery, and the general smell of the J building—Cardiology & Vascular Medicine— at Cleveland Clinic.

The Adult Congenital Heart Association has a website (www.achaheart.org) and a variety of helpful information and links contained within. I began to read the message board. I've read many different message boards in the past, typically triathlon related, but this message board is different. It's very active (with over 1000 members), it's relevant, and I feel a strange sense of comfort and reassurance when I am logged on and reading the postings. I've learned quickly that my condition seems far less complicated than others who have multiple types of defects and have had multiple open-heart surgeries. *Will I need more surgeries?* I wonder. I've also learned some other interesting facts, most recently that there is now research surrounding the connection between an enlarged right side of the heart and a person's intolerance to heat. Despite living many years in the hot and humid climate of Bermuda, Hawaii, and now 18 months in the hot desert climate of Vegas, I have never felt comfortable in extreme heat. I sweat more than the average person, and at night, I have the A/C cranked high enough to cause Don to contemplate wearing a woolen hat to stop shivering. It makes sense; if the heart is less efficient and less able to pump blood around the body, then the blood cannot get to the surface of the skin to perform its cooling function in hot environments. I'm not sure what, if anything, this means for me. Clearly, training in Vegas and racing long-distance endurance events will raise my core temperature to an intolerable level…I may need to consider more elaborate cooling mechanisms and so, of course, I add this to my list of questions for my cardiologist.

Seeing the signs for the clinic gives me a sense of relaxation and comfort. I am happy to be back here, even though the memories of my surgery are powerful and seem like yesterday. The hotel staff greet us at check-in. "Welcome back," they say with caution. What is the polite greeting for a returning patient to the clinic? Don and I joke once again about this dilemma that the hotel staff must face each day.

The next day, I wake in the hotel room and then head to the gym for a treadmill run. Today I run seven miles, and I feel good; the pace is steady, and I am pleased with the workout.

Day one of my tests consists of an echo stress test and blood work. I am once again donning a hospital gown with the clinic's logo printed on the pocket. I feel my heart start to flutter again, and I mention this to the technician. She assures me the readings from the EKG are fine. I am asked to lie down on my left side with my arm above my head. This is my fourth echocardiogram, so I know the routine. The technician places the probe on my left chest and begins the ultrasound. I hear my heart beating through the systems speakers; it sounds irregular to me, but what do I know? The technician is thorough, and I am cold, lying there. A nurse is paged and arrives to administer a saline IV so they can track the bubbles into my heart and see if any bubbles move across the chambers. This is, logically, called a bubble study. The first nurse asks me which arm to place the IV in. I tell her the left is better but I'm still a tough stick. She struggles and cannot find a vein. She gives up and apologizes and pages a more-experienced nurse. He arrives but also has problems. His hands are cold, and I'm now shivering. Finally, he believes he is in. The technician signals him to pump the saline into my vein. This action causes intense pain in my arm. I know it shouldn't, and I scream and swear out loud. They are unsure but assume the vein was pierced in error. Tears roll down my cheeks, and they realize my complaint is not exaggerated. The study is incomplete; there are not enough bubbles in my heart to see the movement, but the nurse withdraws the IV, and the pain subsides. The technician speaks to the radiologist to determine if the study will suffice. They don't stick me again, so I presume it will, thank goodness.

My resting heart rate before the IV was 44 bpm. During the pain, it rose to 70 bpm while still lying flat. The other technician asks me to stand on the treadmill so she can begin the stress test and the readings (EKGs and blood pressure). She increases the incline and the speed over three-minute intervals, and my perceived exertion increases rapidly because of this. My legs feel heavy, tired from my earlier morning run. The technicians laugh about how the machine will eventually beat me and I will beg for surrender. I have no doubt. After ten minutes or so, I have reached 96% of my max heart rate according to their charts. I figure they have just used the standard 220 less my age calculation to result in a max heart rate of 179. I know it is higher than this for me, but today when I reach 171 on the treadmill, I am ready to stop and tell them my perceived exertion is high. Immediately, I am ushered back onto the bed and asked to lie back again for a repeat echo. My heart is pounding. The entire test takes 90 minutes. The technician tells me my right heart chambers are still enlarged but the repair looks good and intact. I am released and head to the lab for a blood draw. Strangely, the nurse has no problem finding a vein on the first attempt, and I am in and out of the lab in four minutes.

I cannot sleep and wake up at 3:30 a.m. Today I see my cardiologist, and I am anxious to learn how my heart is doing. I try not to be optimistic; it has been only three months, and it is likely my heart is still healing. I head to the hotel gym and spin on the stationary bike for an hour. My head is spinning, but my exercise heart rate is steady.

I check in at desk J2-4. Three months ago, I was on the fifth floor, almost immediately above in my hospital room. The smells in the hospital are not unpleasant but familiar and invoke vivid memories. Four other patients are waiting for appointments. All are older than I, and all look unhealthy; two carry oxygen tanks with them. I am checked in and my vital signs taken. The physician's assistant also orders an EKG. Once again, I wear the green gown. I then wait 60 minutes for my cardiologist to arrive. I am told he has had to perform an emergency procedure to close a patient's hole. I wait. His secretary knocks on my door and enters to greet me. I have had many phone conversations with her and am delighted to meet her finally. The feeling is mutual, I think.

Finally, my cardiologist arrives. He seems a little flustered but shares with me his excitement about my echo results. He tells me he is very pleased with how well my heart is doing and says although it is still slightly enlarged, it looks almost normal and functions well under stress. I am not expecting this news and therefore almost can't believe the words I am hearing. He pulls up the images to show me and then compares them with the pre-surgery echo. It is true the right ventricle has shrunk. How miraculous. My right atrium is still enlarged and may never decrease, so he tells me, but this is not concerning him. He then examines me and tells me that all is good and I can resume more intense training. When I question him about racing, however, he is not excited about the Ironman and tells me that "common sense" would lead me to not competing. My heart is still likely healing, and putting it under this much stress may not be wise, although medically there is nothing indicating that it couldn't cope. We agree to compromise and conclude that I will increase my training but check back with him after a couple of months of increased training, and we both remain open-minded to my participation. I am happy with the plan. He tells me to listen to my body: if I feel "crappy," back off. I tell him my vision has been crystal clear on my four-hour bike rides since the surgery. He doesn't seem surprised by this.

We discuss the flutters I feel, and he is not concerned but orders a 24-hour Holter monitor for me to wear at the clinic and hotel so they can monitor my heart rhythms and hopefully rule out any arrhythmia. He tells me his wife has PVCs (premature ventricular contractions) regularly and he is often listening to her heartbeat to reassure her that everything is fine. I ask him my list of questions. He is surprised that I haven't told my parents of my surgery but understands the decision I made. He confirms that my brother and my parents have a 3% chance rather than a 1% chance of having a congenital heart disorder. Still a 97% chance that they do not. He recommends my brother have an echo. At the close of our hour-long meeting, we agree that I will call him in a couple of months to discuss my progress and make a decision about the race and that if all is well, I will see him in a year.

I am fitted with the monitor. The adhesive tabs irritate my skin, but I know it's only for 24 hours, so I will try to ignore it. I can't shower during this time and I am to diarize any symptoms. I make five entries into the diary for times when I feel my heart fluttering.

Linda from executive patient services calls to find out how the tests went; I tell her the good news. She is pleased but secretly sad that we will hopefully not be back anytime soon. I tell her I will mention her in my book.

I am sitting on the plane back to Vegas. Don is in the seat next to me, asleep. This time I am definitely uneasy leaving the clinic. In his physical, the doctors searched hard to find something wrong with him but concluded that he is healthy and fit, one less thing for us to worry about. I am still an open case, but I feel almost discharged again. I wish I lived nearer to Cleveland, or that my Vegas cardiologist was a specialist in adult congenital disorders. I feel special in Cleveland, and in good hands.

CHAPTER 8

The Serious Training Begins: The First Eight Weeks

July 2010

Having received my cardiologist's blessing to increase my training load, I discuss the next two months' plan with my swim coach when I return from Cleveland. His initial approach is aggressive, and I am far from confident that I can achieve this. The time commitment is going to be too much even for me, so we revise the schedule, which still involves a heavy weekly training load. I know that I will have to plan my work schedule very carefully if I am to achieve this. We also discuss my planned two-week vacation to Europe and a realistic adjustment for these weeks in mid-August.

This July is blisteringly hot in Vegas, often topping 110 degrees, hotter than the previous year, and running outside becomes impossible, so I have to quickly become friends with the indoor treadmill. This, though painfully dull, is more manageable and also softer on my knees. I am impressed with my run progression, and I can increase my mileage according to my training plan within the first few weeks. I am also pleased with how well my knees are holding up; the nagging pain from before the knee surgery is no longer present. I am up to eight miles by the end of July for my long run. Only another 18 miles to go!

My typical weekend training includes a lake swim with the triathlon swim group. I am pleased that I am able to reestablish myself in the lead group. One of my fellow swimmers (Dougal) is also signed up to race Ironman Arizona and, coincidentally, our swim abilities are quite similar. The last weekend of July, I wear my wetsuit to get used to swimming in it in preparation for the race. The water temperature is 80 degrees, but the air temperature is ridiculously hot at 115 degrees. I almost melt in the wetsuit and struggle to keep my core temperature down.

The heat also affects my riding. Either I am more intolerant after my heart surgery or this summer is particularly brutal. By 6:00 a.m., the air temperature is already above 90 degrees. I have to fine-tune my hydration on my long rides. I come up with a workable plan, which includes, in part, riding on my indoor trainer in the air-conditioning with a fan blowing directly onto my head. Even with this, the sweat continually drips off my chin. By the end of July, my long rides are approximately seventy miles in length. Given the ever-present wind in Las Vegas and the hilly terrain, a 70-mile ride is already a four-hour ride. I feel strong, though, and my heart rate is good. I am gaining noticeable strength and fitness every day.

I have two additional medical appointments scheduled in Vegas before I leave for vacation. The first is with my local cardiologist. I am once again thoroughly examined and given an EKG. I provide copies of my Cleveland medical reports and a disc with my latest echo. My cardiologist is very pleased with my progress but seems to have no comprehension of the level of training I am currently doing. I try to explain and ask if it is too much, but he assures me that exercise is the best thing I can do. We also discuss my heart flutters, and I tell him I have seen a pattern with caffeine and alcohol. He confirms that these two vices can cause changes in a heartbeat and that he is not surprised. He explains that my heart is likely a little more sensitive. It is a condition known as "holiday heart." Seemingly, the holiday indulgences can often result in arrhythmia and heart conditions. He cautions me to reduce my caffeine intake and allows me the occasional glass of wine. Coffee is one of my favorite things of all time, so I frantically scour the local grocery stores to obtain some high-quality espresso-style decaffeinated coffee! He tells me he wants to see me in six months, at which time he will schedule another echo. He is confident there will be no further complications.

Next up is my appointment with my primary care physician. It's been two months since I last saw her, and I am excited to demonstrate how well I am doing. The nurse takes my vital signs and tells me that my doctor will be happy to see me doing so well. We discuss the Cleveland trip and also talk about my Ironman intentions. Once an avid tennis player, my doctor understands the athletic urge that I have to compete, although she asks if I have the willpower to hold back and not let my heart rule my head. The irony of this statement. I'm not sure of the answer to this yet, and I need to give it some serious thought before I commit. She is very pleased with my progress, and for the first time in four months, she does not request that I schedule a follow-up. I feel happy but almost a little anxious that my regular visits are now over.

It is July 29, my last day before we take off on a two-and-a-half–week vacation to Europe. This past week has been an intense training week consisting of more than 16 kilometers of swimming, more than 20 miles of running, and more than 260 miles of cycling. I am utterly exhausted and cannot wait to take a well-earned break. Today, I receive an e-mail from the race director at Ironman Arizona.

> ..... You may already know, there was recently a dam breach in Tempe Lake, which serves as the swim venue for the Ford Ironman Arizona Triathlon. We recognize your concern as a registered athlete for the event. The Ironman Team continues to closely monitor the situation and its impact to the Tempe Town Lake area, and is currently working with the City of Tempe and local agencies. Our team remains committed to providing an Ironman experience that includes swim, bike and run.

I'm certainly not sure what to make of this. I guess there is a possibility that the dam will not be fixed and that the race will not have a swim portion. Because the swim is my strongest discipline, I would not be willing to compete without it. I have mixed feelings about this; part of me is concerned that I may not be able to compete, but the other part of me is happy to let fate take its course, and if the race is cancelled, then so be it, my Ironman dream will be postponed until 2011.

I also receive an e-mail from my surgeon asking if Don and I would like to be a part of the Cleveland Clinic running and triathlon team. He is trying to put together a team of former patients and physicians to compete in a race in Cleveland or NYC. I don't hesitate to respond and tell him that we would be delighted to!

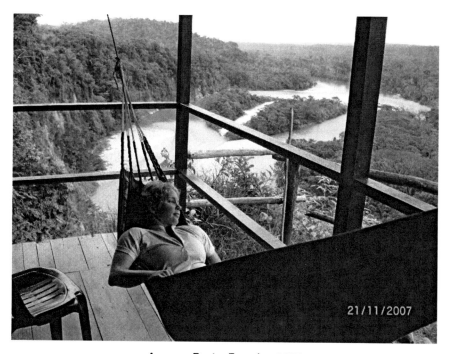

Amazon Basin, Ecuador, 2007

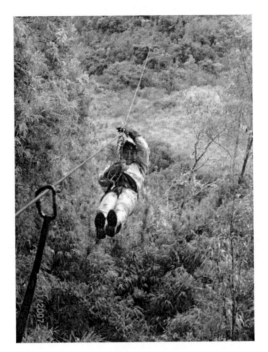

Zip-lining

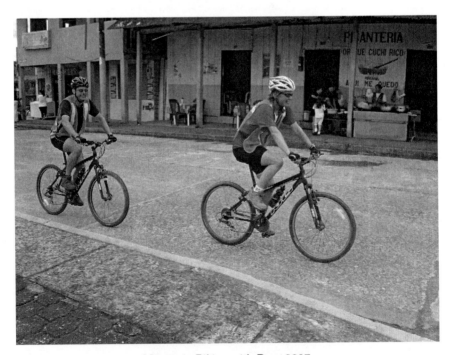

Mountain Biking with Don, 2007

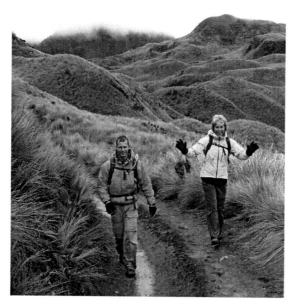

Hiking in the Andes, 2007

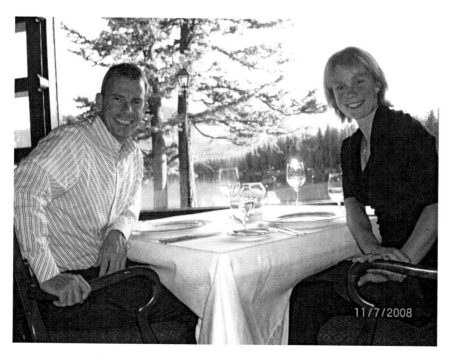

Living Life to the full, Jasper National Park 2008

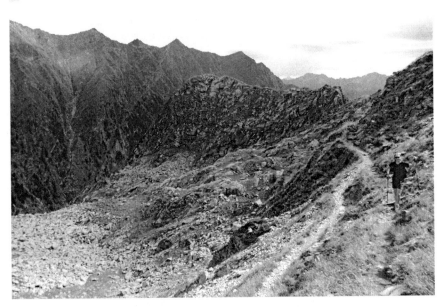

Hiking Northern Italy, Summer 2010, 5 months post surgery

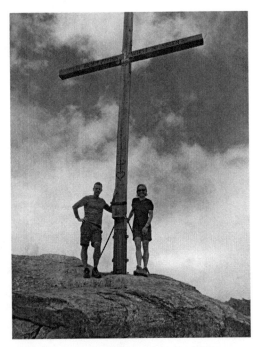

Italian Mountain peak, 9000 feet, 5 months post surgery

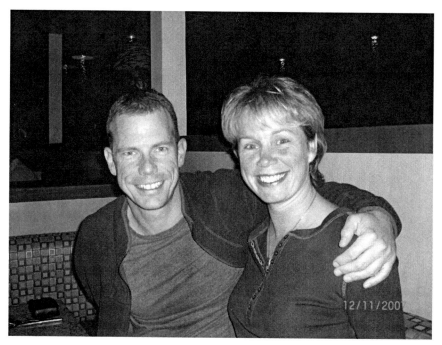

My Husband, best friend and soul mate

CHAPTER 9

Vacation in Europe

August 2010

In January we had planned a trip to Peru, with the aim to climb up to Machu Picchu. During that first phone conversation with the doctor from Cleveland, I had asked if I would have time in June to take a vacation or whether it was possible I would be undergoing treatment for the suspected vasculitis. He had suggested that a short vacation would be fine, but he specifically said, "No high altitudes, no Machu Picchu." I hadn't even mentioned our plans to him at that point! June came and went, and the only trip we made, of course, was back to Cleveland. This August, however, my cousin was to be married, so Don and I had planned our vacation around this event, also including mountains, cities, friends, and family.

This will also be the trip when I will tell my parents about the past five months of my life.

The last leg of our fabulous vacation has arrived all too soon, and we are flying back from Prague to London. We have had a fun-packed time and, of course, a very active one. In fact, my training was fairly solid, perhaps not as intense, but definitely regular and disciplined. We included some cross-training activities such as mountain biking and hiking in the Alps, all truly fantastic. I'm confident that I did the best I could to maintain my fitness level.

The final leg of our vacation is my cousin's wedding. The night before the wedding, I will recount my story to my parents. I am still very unsure whether this is the right thing to do and how I will begin. Don and I decide that we will just wait for the moment; he is confident that I will know when that is.

My mum is waiting for me and staring out of the window as we drive up to their apartment building. She is overwhelmed to see us, overjoyed, in fact, after two years since our last visit. The feeling is mutual, but I am instantly apprehensive about telling her and creating so much unhappiness and worry for them both. I push the inevitable conversation to later in the evening after a jovial dinner and chat for a few hours. Almost five months have passed, and I still don't know how to begin the conversation. I am hoping for an opening, something in our conversation that is a natural lead-in. My mum begins to tell us that she is reading a book called *The Secret*. I know of this book; it is a motivational-style book and is based around positive thinking. My heart quickens and my palms sweat as I know now that this is my moment. I ask her if she has changed her behavior as a result of reading the book. She replies that she is trying to think more positively and trying not to worry as much about things.

I begin my story by starting at the end.

The overwhelming release of pressure lifts once I have begun, and now I cannot control the emotional tears that roll down my face. I turn to Don, and he reassures me that everything is fine and encourages me to continue. I quickly gather myself and do just that, detail by detail.

My parents sit in silence and are clearly in shock. They ask few questions; even without much discussion, my story takes the better part of two hours to tell. I decide to explain as many details as I can in the hope that the more information I can provide, the more I can educate and therefore replace their fear with knowledge. But that is too much to expect. I look at their faces as I explain the details of the ICU, and my dad places his head in his hands. My mum holds back her tears and is speechless.

Don and I focus on the positives and end the conversation on these aspects, of which there are many. Lying in bed after midnight, I wonder if my decision was the right one. I certainly don't feel any better by telling them, and I'm absolutely sure I have ruined what they were hoping would be a wonderful family reunion weekend.

I was naïve to think that my cousin's wedding would extinguish the pain they would feel. I reassure myself that honesty is still the best principle.

I haven't yet seen my brother, Paul, who lives close to my parents. We haven't seen each other for three years, yet I feel like we are so much closer since we've shared parts of this journey together over the phone. It is wonderful to finally see him, and when we embrace for the first time, there is so much communication between us without any words spoken. He promises to help my parents through the next phase as they try to rationalize and understand. He and I, however, clearly underestimate the benefit of time that we have both had and underestimate how much time our parents will both need.

It is time to say good-bye and journey home to Las Vegas. I am determined to be strong, yet seeing my mum so upset makes it hard for me to hold back my tears. I am saddened that I have caused them so much stress.

CHAPTER 10

Doubts and Reassurance

September 2010

A m I insane? Do I seriously think I can compete in an Ironman race just eight months after open-heart surgery? I'm starting to have some serious doubts, about not only whether I will physically be able to complete the 140.6 miles but, more importantly, whether this will be reckless and damage my newly fixed heart, perhaps even send me back to the operating room. I'm starting to lose my focus, and my training has started to suffer. I tell myself that it doesn't really matter because I probably will not end up doing the race. But what causes the stress for me is not being able to make a decision. I don't feel sufficiently medically informed to know all the risks and consequences. I decide to contact my friend, and founder of the Ironheart Racing team, Dave. Like me, he's a triathlete with a heart defect or two, and I know he will help me make some choices.

Dave instantly recommends I make an appointment with his congenital heart cardiologist in Seattle. He tells me that she just "gets it" and, one way or the other, will direct me. To race or not to race, that is the question.

I call the hospital at the University of Washington and schedule an appointment for two weeks' time. Already, I feel relieved that now the decision will be somewhat out of my hands.

On September 15, I fly to Seattle for two days to meet with Dr. Karen Stout and her team. Dr. Stout heads up the Adult Congenital Heart

Program at the University of Washington Heart Center. She spends several hours with me, and I'm delighted with her level of detail, thoroughness, and no-nonsense direction. I have never doubted the medical opinions and excellent care that I have received to date in either Vegas or Cleveland, but recently I have needed just a little something more, a doctor who understands my drive to compete in the Ironman event and yet is sufficiently knowledgeable about my condition to educate me and direct me on the risks and limitations. I have been looking for a medical partner, someone whom I could, hopefully, rely on from here on in and someone who was accessible physically and remotely. Dr. Stout fits perfectly into this role for me, and I am delighted that I am now one of her patients.

The hospital in Seattle brings back some vivid memories, of course. I'm sure that I will always have these feelings whenever I visit a hospital from here on in. Strangely, however, on this visit, I don't feel like a patient but more like a visitor. My primary purpose for this trip is to obtain a medical determination on whether or not to race in the Ironman. Dr. Stout evaluates me and has me undergo a series of tests, all of which I have previously done at some point in Cleveland, but now it is several months later. I spend more than an hour with her discussing my condition, my training, my recovery, my current pains, my potential risks and limitations. She orders a cardiac MRI, a treadmill stress test, an echocardiogram, and, of course, an EKG. She explains that her main concern is whether my right ventricle has reduced in size sufficiently since the surgery. She considers this primary fact the main guide as to whether I should race. An enlarged right ventricle represents a compromised heart, and a compromised heart powering me through an Ironman could potentially fail on me.

Lying in the MRI chamber again, I am as claustrophobic as I was during the test in Cleveland. It's hard to relax when you can see no further than a couple of inches above your head and when any movement is restricted, in fact forbidden. Although not physically painful, the cardiac MRI is most unpleasant for these reasons, and I know I will have to undergo this test many more times in my life, as this is the best way to gain an accurate reading of the size of my right ventricle.

I also have the pleasure of wearing a new style of gown, with an opening at the front rather than the back, thankfully. The echo is relatively unremarkable; this is the sixth echo I have had in six months. The treadmill stress test is also similar to the test I had done in Cleveland a few months earlier, but this time, I am able to achieve a maximum heart rate of 183 before I beg for mercy.

I meet with Dr. Stout again following the results of the tests, and she shares with me her views and the findings. The MRI shows a significant reduction in right ventricle size. Pre-surgery, the size units were 220, compared to a reading of 130 now. She is pleased with this reduction and all of the other test results and concludes that there is nothing medically indicating that I cannot participate in the race. We do, however, discuss some conditions that I need to be mindful of. Should they occur, I should consider not racing:

1. My training and racing heart rate should, on average, stay beneath 160 bpm. This will mean no very hard interval training. I will not be racing by my power meter or by the clock but rather by my heart rate.
2. If the recent chest pain returns and persists, she would not recommend competing this year. She explains that the pain was likely musculoskeletal and unlikely to be heart related but that it is possibly related to the pericarditus that I experienced during my initial recovery weeks, in which case, no race.
3. If I experience any abnormal heart rhythms when training— either accelerated or skipped beats—she will order a monitor for me to wear again and evaluate whether this is anything significant, perhaps an arrhythmia, in which case, no race.

I am to let her know how the next few weeks of training progress. Fingers crossed, I would make it to the start line.

I'm mildly confident as I journey back to Vegas and prepare to adapt my training plan accordingly, replacing the very intense sessions with moderately hard workouts that will ensure my heart rate does not exceed 160 bpm. I'm happy that I have a plan and a doctor who really does "get it."

Within the first week of being back, I train and notice that during a run, my heart rate spikes, unusually so. I'm concerned that after just a few days, I am e-mailing my doctor about this, but I know that is what I must do. True to her parting words, she responds quickly by e-mail, and we develop a plan to monitor the next few training runs. She suspects this is nothing significant, and the fact that I picked up a cold most likely affected my run. There are no recurring issues in the coming weeks.

CHAPTER 11

My First Race

October 2010

It has been almost 11 months since my last race. Today, I will compete in an open-water swim at Lake Mead. It is the inaugural Slam the Dam race and has been organized by the local triathlon-swimming club, Swim Las Vegas. The temperature of the lake is still relatively warm at this time of year, and many competitors choose not to wear a wetsuit. I want to practice in my wetsuit, however, as I know I will be wearing one in seven weeks in Arizona. The distance I will swim will be 2.4 miles. I've only ever raced this distance once before, at the Silverman Triathlon, 11 months ago. At the time, I was swimming faster and more consistently than I have been recently, and I'm still a little behind where I would like to be in my training by this point. Still, it is what it is, and it will be good to go through the pre-race routine and get in the race practice. I've chosen not to do any other triathlon races before the Ironman; perhaps this isn't wise, but I wanted to protect my knees in particular from the strain that comes with racing and save that for November 21.

The gun goes off, and I stumble on the rocky beach beneath me, but I am quickly swimming straight for the first buoy. Hands, arms, and feet are all jostling for position, as is always the case in an open-water swim, a mad scramble at the start. After I make the first turn, I try to settle in to a steady rhythm. I know I must do this, as I have at least an hour of swimming ahead of me and I will surely run out of steam unless I get my pace under control. I find a pair of feet ahead of me and try to stay behind them. There is an advantage from drafting behind someone swimming in front of you: your effort is reduced, yet you maintain the same speed. Unfortunately, the swimmer ahead of me is not swimming very straight, and the additional back and forth is causing me to veer in the wrong direction, so I resume my own position and head for the next buoy.

The course is a T shape, and the back stretch of the T seems to take forever to complete. My pacing must be off, either that or my fitness isn't where I was expecting it to be, as I am struggling to stay strong and I know my speed must have reduced. My wetsuit is heating up, and it is too hot to be swimming an hour at this intensity in a wet suit. The air temperature and the water temperature are the same at 80 degrees. Finally, I make the finally turn and head for the shore. I try to increase my pace, but my arms have other plans, and the heat in my shoulders causes them to rebel. I cross the finish line in a time of 1 hour and 3 minutes, just 4 minutes slower than 11 months ago. I am pleased with the time but not in how I feel; the effort was greater than I was hoping to have to do to achieve that time, and I know I have to lower my expectations and my speed for the Ironman race, as I still will have 112 miles to cycle and 26.2 miles to run! My swim coach congratulates me, as I have finished first in my division. Swimming has always been my strength, so this is no major surprise, but still after everything I have been through, this is a great result for my first race back.

Six weeks to go until the Ironman. My training is going well; I have no more heart palpitations, no more chest pain, and my endurance is definitely increasing. I feel I am on track and that getting to the start line is very achievable.

 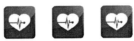

I had never experienced an injury until I turned 35. I guess that was officially the end of my youth. My first injury was as a result of playing soccer in Hawaii for a recreational women's team. I aggressively reached for a moving ball and as a result pulled my hamstring. I'm not sure I really knew how to treat it at the time; I certainly didn't apply the RICE treatment that I so readily do today. RICE stands for rest, ice, compression, and elevation, an athlete's mantra. This hamstring injury prevented me from running for three weeks, which seems nothing to me now, but at the time, I was running six days a week, and I felt my athletic endeavors had come to an abrupt end.

I'm not sure I remember how I made the decision then to seek out a masters swim class, but nonetheless I did and found myself entering the Nuuanu Masters Swim class at the YMCA that next week. Swimming was the only exercise that didn't aggravate my hamstring injury. I hadn't swam seriously since the age of 15; now, more than 20 years later, I was apprehensive as I stood on the pool deck and introduced myself to Coach Mark. Mark has coached at the YMCA for over thirty years; he has dedicated his time and experience to hundreds of adult swimmers and has not taken a penny for his services. Mark is a true testament to Hawaii's Aloha spirit, and he welcomed me with open arms. The language and style of swimming had changed significantly in the past 20 years, and I realized I needed to quickly learn many of the basics such as circle swimming, flip turns (again), and work-out abbreviations. What exactly is a negative split or a descending set? I remember that first workout in which I swam for an hour; I was so exhausted at the end of the work-out I could barely drive home. I doubt we swam more than two thousand meters, but that first workout will always stick in my memory as the entry into my triathlon world. I loved swimming with this group and joined them twice a week and sometimes on the weekend for an ocean swim along the Waikiki shoreline. These ocean swims were heavenly, and I now look forward to my visits to Hawaii so I can swim with the honus (the Hawaiian name for turtles) and enjoy the spirit of Aloha again and again.

I never really considered training for a triathlon until a fellow swimmer at the masters class suggested it to me. I had purchased a road bike in San Francisco but had barely ridden it, but something stirred inside me, and I began researching online for beginner triathlon clubs. Fortunately, Hawaii is riddled with such clubs, and I soon found myself joining in a mini-tri as my first triathlon experience. We had to swim approximately two hundred yards along the shorefront, then cycle no more than ten miles before finishing with a run around Kapiolani Park, which was maybe three kilometers. Staggeringly, I was one of the first women to finish, and a few raised eyebrows were shot at me. Who was this girl who simply showed up and swam like fish, biked like a veteran, and ran like a scared rabbit? I joined the club that very day, and TeamJet has ever since been a part of my life. When I visit Hawaii, I make an effort to join their training rides or runs and say Aloha.

My hamstring injury was annoying and took many months to finally heal. I ended up seeing a sports doctor at the Queens medical facility in Honolulu and experienced my first ever cortisone shot, at the very top of my hamstring, a shot in the butt, so to speak.

Once you experience an injury, other injuries often plague you as your body becomes imbalanced and tries to overcompensate. Next came a stress fracture in my foot that sidelined me from everything for a couple of months and resulted in me having to wear a removable boot for six weeks. Whilst the stress fracture occurred in Hawaii, it wasn't until we had moved back to Bermuda that it was diagnosed and treated. Once I was allowed to remove the boot, I underwent three months of physical therapy with my therapist, Dee, who has since become a very close friend and fellow triathlete. Dee nursed me back to fitness and not only treated my stress fracture but continued to work on other injuries that plagued me.

After a significantly hilly trail run in Vermont in the summer of 2007, I felt a sharp pain in the side of my knee. My knees had never bothered me before, but that day marked the beginning of three years of knee injuries. Iliotibial band syndrome, or ITB pain, is a common triathlete injury. The ITB is a band of tissue that runs along the outside of the thigh and connects the hip to the knee. As this tightens and shortens, it causes friction at the two attachment points, which can result in inflammation and significant knife-like, sharp pain. Over the course of the next two years, I suffered this injury in both knees and became somewhat of a guru in the necessary treatment. Gone were the days when I could simply lace up my running shoes and head out for a 40-minute run and be back at work, showered and changed, an hour later. Now there was significant stretching, icing, leg exercises, and even rolling on a foam roller to loosen the ITB before and after exercise. A 40-minute run had turned in to a 90-minute exercise. Still, it had to be done if I wanted to still train and compete. I remember arriving at the World Half Ironman Championships in Florida in 2007, praying that my knee would let me run the half marathon at the end of the race. After just three miles, the stabbing pain returned, and I ran the next 10 miles in agony. Still, I ran through that finishing tape and experienced that amazing sense of accomplishment. My next few months were all about healing.

I've also suffered runner's knee, a condition in which the kneecap over time becomes misaligned and incorrectly tracks over the rest of the knee joint, causing pain as the cartilage gradually wears away. I have become proficient at various taping techniques to hold my kneecaps in place. My knee injuries have prevented me from entering and training for a full marathon, which, at times, has been disappointing.

Just six weeks before race day, I am somewhat injury free. I have a slight Achilles tendonitis, perhaps from new running shoes or hiking up a mountain in Italy in August. It is not, thankfully, preventing me from progressing through my run training, and I am now up to 16 miles for my long runs. This is the longest I have ever run, and I'm pretty excited about it. Don now calls my long runs Charnley World Records, as each week, I run farther than I have ever run before.

On October 16, I enter another race, a charity century ride around Las Vegas. Viva Bike Vegas is an annual event, and this year, the route is a spectacular 115 miles, including a section over the new bridge (yet to be open to traffic) over Lake Mead and overlooking the Hoover Dam. I decide to test my strength a little and push myself a little harder than I would normally do on one of my long rides. I am pleased with my result on this hilly course and also am able to run for an hour immediately after finishing the ride. It is a very memorable day and also a great day of training with Dougal.

CHAPTER 12

The Final Training Weeks

October 2010

I t's not ideal five weeks before the race, but this next week, I have
another business trip to Hawaii. I receive nothing more than a heav-
enward look and a roll of the eyes from friends when I say I *have* to go to
Hawaii for 10 days. Fair enough, I would be somewhat envious and skeptical that it was a potential hardship if I were hearing someone tell me this.
Regardless, the travel, the client meetings, and the hectic schedule all
point towards very little time for training and, most likely, little sleep. I
must to do the best I can, however. I will borrow a friend's bike and make
sure I at least get in a long ride on the weekend. In addition, there is a
local running race that is 30 kilometers. This will again mark the longest
I have ever run, and I am looking forward to the challenge. I am a little
concerned about the heat and humidity, but, hopefully, the 5:00 a.m. start
time will make it cool enough to allow me to jog my way through it.

My training load was heavy the weekend prior to my trip and consisted
of a 90-minute open-water swim in Lake Mead, followed by a hilly 2-
hour ride on Saturday, then a 110-mile ride on Sunday followed by an
hour-long jog immediately following the bike ride. I was determined to
put in a solid effort because of my upcoming travel and potentially
reduced training; however, my immune system was struggling and I
developed my second cold in three weeks. As a result, I headed straight
to the doctor on Monday to get a flu shot and some antibiotics. Getting sick was not an option for me; I needed my strength at full throt-
tle not only for my training but also for the travel and the busy work
schedule in Hawaii.

For the past few weeks, my training has occupied somewhere from 20 to 25 hours per week. Given this volume, I've had little time for anything other than work and sleep. Don has been so busy at the hotel that he is thankful I have had something occupying my time.

I have been checking the news reports regularly in Tempe, Arizona, to see if there has been any progress on the repair of the lake dam. Surprisingly, the repair work was completed by early October and the gates opened to begin filling the lake. It was anticipated that the lake would be completely full two weeks ahead of schedule, by early November, and therefore the race would go ahead as planned on the existing course. This was a relief. The temperature of the water, however, surely has to be much colder than in prior years. Apparently, the previous year, some competitors found the cold water temperature unbearable, requiring warming blankets after they completed the swim. There are some things you can prepare for and others that you cannot, and swimming in cold water in the late summer in Las Vegas is not an easy thing to do. Still, I made a note to take an extra swim cap with me to Tempe, as wearing two swim caps can provide that much-needed insulation against rapid heat loss.

My 10 days in Hawaii are as busy as I expected them to be, with many client meetings, a conference, and several client dinners. Still, I am able to train every day in some form or another. The duration and intensity is definitely reduced, but at least my frequency stays moderately consistent. The highlights of my trip are the ocean swims, the 60 mile ride with my good friend Steve and the 30k running race. Swimming at the Ala Moana beach park is fantastic. It is a sheltered inlet of the ocean with buoys every 250 meters, so mapping out a 4-kilometer swim was simple. Swimming without a wetsuit is wonderful, and there is always something wonderful to look at Ala Moana. I envy the swimmers in Hawaii who get to do this each week.

At 5:00 a.m. on October 24, I set off on my first running race in many years. I seriously do not remember the last time I entered a running race. It was so much easier getting ready for this race without having to deal with my bike or swimming gear. It is hot and humid, however, at 5:00 a.m., and I am concerned about whether I will be able to run the whole 18.6 miles, so I conservatively set off at a very slow jog, along with many of the other 1000 entrants, one of them my great friend, Debbie. It is a great atmosphere, and I am enjoying seeing the mile markers pass by, one by one. My heart rate is in zone 1 or 2 the whole time, and I am very pleased with my pacing. At the turnaround point, I feel so great that I start to pick up the pace, and before I know it, I am passing several people who started the race too fast. Note to self: remember this in four weeks' time; slow and steady may not win the race but hopefully will mean I can finish! As I run down the finishing stretch, I am ecstatic; this is the longest I have ever run, and I feel great. I have completed the 30k in a time of three hours and six minutes and still have plenty of gas left in the tank. It's another Charnley world record! That is an average of 10 minutes per mile. Certainly, there is no award for speed for me, but I am still able to come 13th out of 60 women in my age group…not bad for my first running race in years. Finishing so strong and running up to the finish line, I smile as I cross the line; I know at this point that I am ready to tackle the Ironman both mentally and physically.

After the race, I meet with Ryan, a fellow member of the Ironheart Racing team, who lives in Hawaii. I have been e-mailing with him over the past couple of months. Ryan and I chat easily for a short while and share heart stories. Ryan is not only an inspiration but also a great athlete. He has competed in countless races in many endurance sports, and if it wasn't for the scar down his chest, you would not know that he has had open-heart surgery or that he suffers from a rare condition in which the pericardium sticks to his heart and calcifies. He will at some point require further surgery again to correct this, but until that point, endurance exercise helps minimize the effects. Talking to a fellow heart-surgery patient is therapeutic and very motivational. I could have chatted with Ryan for many hours, but time runs away with us both, and we say good-bye with a hug; he wishes me well and says he'll be cheering for me.

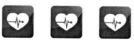

Some say that the Ironman event is the single most grueling endurance event that exists. Triathlon was first developed in Southern California in the 1970s, so it is a relatively young sport. Its popularity has grown exponentially over the past few decades, particularly since the 2000 Olympics, when triathlon became an Olympic sport.

There are several different distances in triathlon, and the rules can also vary slightly, depending on whether the race is professional or amateur. The sprint distance is, as the name suggests, the shortest of the triathlons. The swim portion of a sprint triathlon is usually between 500 and 800 meters long, the bike portion is approximately 25 kilometers, and the run is 5 kilometers. Sprint-distance triathlons are common events for beginners, and the training involved to prepare for one is much less than for some of the longer-distance triathlons. During my early years in Hawaii, I entered a number of sprint-distance races and learned the basics of the sport without having to commit endless hours to training. Sprint distances are fast races, and I think my fast days are most likely behind me now, but they are definitely fun and involve the whole community.

The intermediate distance became known as the Olympic-distance triathlon after the 2000 Olympics. This distance includes a 1500-meter swim, a 40-kilometer bike ride, and a 10-kilometer run. For professional athletes, this distance is raced throughout the world as part of the Triathlon World Cup and culminates with the World Championships once a year in a designated country. In 2006, the World Championships were held in Lausanne, Switzerland. The professional event is a "drafting" event. Drafting is described as riding close behind another rider, therefore being shielded from the wind, which results in a significantly reduced effort for the rider behind. Professional triathletes performing this distance in these races are permitted to draft; therefore, the bike portion is more akin to a bicycle race, so the fastest runner often then wins the triathlon. At most World Cup races, including the World Championships, there is amateur race. In 2006, I was a resident in Bermuda and represented Bermuda at the amateur World Championships in Lausanne. This was an amazing experience and one I shall never forget.

I competed with the best amateurs in the world and enjoyed every minute. Unknown to me at the time, not only did I have a congenital heart defect but I was also suffering from a stress fracture in my foot.

Both sprint- and Olympic-distance triathlons are deemed short-course triathlons. Long-course distances consist of the half Ironman and the full Ironman. The half Ironman consists of a 1.2-mile swim, a 56-mile bike ride, and a 13.2-mile run (a half marathon). Training for a half Ironman takes significantly more effort and time than training for short-course racing. To date, I have completed five half Ironmans. Each of them has given me a tremendous sense of accomplishment. My times for completing this distance have been relatively competitive for my age group, my fastest time being 5 hours and 18 minutes at the World Championships in Clearwater, Florida, in 2007. The swim portion of the race is always a nerve-wracking start, but once that's completed, it's possible to settle down into a steady rhythm on the bike and start to enjoy the day. Training for the half marathon portion has always been a challenge for me because of various injuries, so I've often struggled through the run portion. The last half Ironman that I raced was in April 2009. I remember getting off the bike and beginning my run portion and thinking, *How am I ever going to run 13.2 miles!* I hope when I finish the bike leg of the Ironman in Arizona, I feel better than that.

It is not only the time training that one needs to invest in to compete in triathlon but also the equipment. It can certainly be an expensive sport. Of course it is possible to complete a triathlon with a swimsuit, a pair of goggles, a standard bicycle, a helmet, and a pair of running shoes, but most participants who compete in long-course events have significantly more equipment than this.

Three weeks to go, and this morning's training is my last long run. My schedule says 20 miles, and I am excited to reach this milestone. The weather in Vegas is now cold in the mornings, and the temperature this morning is only 50 degrees. I am running this morning according to my race-day marathon plan, which is to run very slowly for the first six miles, then increase the speed gradually with the hope of running what is termed a negative split, whereby the second half of the run is faster than the first half. I carry my water with me in a belt around my waist. I am wearing my race-day outfit and plan to consume energy gels every hour. I start the run. The air is cold; I enjoy running in the cooler weather. It is 5:30 a.m. and still dark outside. My chosen route runs north-south rather than east-west, which will result in fewer hills and therefore simulate the course in Arizona. I run successfully according to the plan, and the miles tick by. By mile 15, I am starting to feel the fatigue, and I take in my final gel. My pace is right on track, and I finish the 20 miles in exactly 3 hours and 20 minutes, therefore averaging 10-minute miles and yet another Charnley world record. I'm delighted with the result; my knees held up. After a recovery breakfast and some well-needed stretching, I am pleased with how I feel. I know I can complete the Ironman.

My final long ride is two days later, and I ride with my training partner and friend Dougal. We ride for six hours across Las Vegas from the Red Rock Mountains down into Henderson. We both feel strong, despite the strong wind that seems to hit at us from every direction. I practice my race-day nutrition and hydration and then quickly transition into my running shoes and jog easily for an hour. At the end of this final hard training week, I have run 50 miles, cycled 200 miles, and swam 6 miles. I am exhausted and looking forward to the three weeks of taper that are ahead.

CHAPTER 13

The Taper and Preparations

November 2010

When I first heard the term "taper" years ago, I had visions of wrapping myself in tape to prevent injuries, perhaps, so close to a race. After training with my first triathlon team in Hawaii, I learned that the taper is actually a period just prior to a race that consists of a reduced training load so as to allow the body to recover from the recent hard training weeks and prepare it for race day. There are many different theories about tapering; some people taper for several weeks, and others just for a few days. The length of the taper typically matches the duration of the race, so for Ironman racing, the taper period can be anywhere from two to four weeks. My training program calls for a three-week taper. Each week, my training volume decreases, first by 40%, then by 60%, and then, in the final week, the number of hours spent training is very minimal, as rest and recovery become the most important drivers. Training intensity, however, still stays relatively high to keep the muscles stimulated and the body loose.

This close to the race, I start to focus my mind whenever I can on race day and start to visualize crossing the finish line. I smile when I imagine the moment, and my eyes fill with an excited tear or two.

My good friends from Bermuda are visiting for a vacation. They have recently completed Ironman Canada and are both very talented athletes. It is fun to train with them during this time. The last time they visited was in April this year, and I was only just one week post surgery so had to watch them ride off without me. This time, the situation is different, and we spend several glorious days riding together. They also provide me with much advice based on their recent Ironman experience. It's a fun two weeks, and having them visit certainly takes my mind off any pre-race stress and anxiety.

Don has developed a head cold, what terrible timing. I increase my vitamin C intake and keep my distance from him. Getting sick is not an option; the Ironman will be tough enough without a cold to contend with also.

Wednesday, November 17 is packing and preparation day; race day is around the corner. Packing for a triathlon is a complicated and detailed affair, and I go through a methodical checklist to make sure that I haven't forgotten anything. One of the reasons I selected Arizona for the venue was because it is driving distance from Las Vegas. This means I don't have to dismantle my bike, pack it in a special bike box, and pay the airline a small fortune to transport it to another state. Instead, I can simply put down the back seats in my mini-SUV and drive with all my additional gear, much simpler.

I have to get not only my race-day gear together but also my nutrition that I will need on the day: gels, bars, and sports drinks. I have practiced consuming this stuff for months, and I shall be glad when I can take a break from these manufactured calories, but for one more day, they will provide me with the appropriate energy that I will need. Over these past eight months, our little dog, Dude, and I have become even more inseparable. I believe that dogs have the ability to know when something isn't quite right with their owners. Dude has been intently protective, and if it were up to him, he would never leave my side, 24 hours a day, 7 days a week. We have decided to take Dude with us; this will be his first road trip, and we are excited to be bringing him along. This, however, means more planning and more packing. Fortunately, we have found a dog-friendly hotel to stay at. I didn't even realize these hotels existed.

We arrive in Tempe, Arizona, three days before the race; this is the perfect time, not too early and not too late. There is much to do before the race, and the race director has published an athlete's guide with a schedule of events to help guide the athletes through the necessary steps in the days leading up to the race.

Once settled in the hotel, we head out to the race site for the first time, just two days before race day. Athlete registration is my first stop. All athletes need to register prior to race day. At registration, I am handed a health waiver to sign. It has been partly completed for me already, and under the box Medical Conditions, my recent open-heart surgery is listed. I pause for a moment and take in a deep breath. Eight months ago, it was impossible to imagine just getting to this point. One of the volunteers checks my details and hands me my race package containing the various numbers (one for the bike, one for my helmet, and one for my tri-top); a timing chip to wear around my ankle, which will record my time at various points along the course; and an information package. She also secures a plastic blue bracelet around my wrist. This confirms I am a registered Ironman competitor and will allow me access into the race site. My volunteer is smiling and seems excited for me; she tells me about the race from her own experiences in prior years. She also asks me if I am nervous about the swim portion. I reply that I'm less nervous about that portion, as I am a confident swimmer, but nevertheless I have never started a race with 2500 other competitors in the water at the same time. She shares with me some advice on where to line up on the starting line to best avoid the mayhem that will undoubtedly be all around me.

We check out the Ironman merchandise for sale; there are so many wonderful items of clothing and gadgets, all containing the M-dot logo. I am somewhat superstitious so refrain from purchasing anything until after the race, lest I should jinx the outcome. I spend the rest of the day resting and hydrating.

Race day minus one, my nerves are starting to mount. This morning is the practice swim. Up until now, athletes have not been permitted to enter the lake for a practice swim. This morning, the race officials have opened up a small part of the lake and will allow all registered athletes to enter the lake for a short swim. I am excited to test out my stroke and to feel the temperature of the lake. I know it will be cool, but I am expecting mid-60s. The race director announces the water temperature: 61 degrees. It will be cold. I jump in and swim to the turn buoy. The water does feel cold, but I swim hard to warm up and soon feel comfortable in the water. My stroke feels strong and relaxed, and I am happy with my short practice swim of 1000 meters. The air temperature has dropped over the past couple of days, and the forecast for race day is cooler still, with increased wind and possible rain. I try not to focus on the weather.

The next stop is at the bike transition field to drop off my bike along with my gear bags, one for the bike and one for the run. I slip my bike onto the rack next to my race number, 2451. The race site is congested; there are athletes everywhere. It can be intimidating, and I can't help but think that everyone looks fitter and faster than me.

All done, we head back to the hotel to rest, eat, and, hopefully, sleep. I cannot believe that tomorrow is the Ironman.

CHAPTER 14

Race Day: The Swim

November 2010

It is 12:57 a.m. November 21, 2010, race-day morning. I have had only three hours' sleep and am lying awake, fighting the rush of thoughts galloping through my mind. What a year it has been, almost eight months to the day since my surgery. I could never have imagined eight months ago that I would be about to embark on one of the greatest days of my life. How can I possibly get back to sleep? My thoughts are just too loud right now. The hotel room is hot; Don and Dude are still sleeping. I get up to use the bathroom, the first of many times, I suspect. I run through my pre-race checklist in my head: fill bottles, tape my knees, smother my body in Vaseline, sprinkle baby powder in my socks, check the pressure in my tires, put my bike into a low gear, etc. I go back to bed and try to relax with some deep breathing. By 3:00 a.m., I decide to get up and have some breakfast. By eating this far before the race start, my stomach will be allowed to fully digest the food and hopefully reduce the chance of stomach issues during the day. My pre-race breakfast is always the same, a bagel with peanut butter and jelly. Of course, I am not remotely hungry and it is a struggle to finish the whole bagel. I go back to bed and lie down for a further hour.

At 4:00 a.m., the alarm bells bleep. Don and Dude stir and we are all finally awake. I make coffee and put on my race gear. I am proud to be wearing the Ironheart Racing Team uniform. I tape my knees carefully with medical tape, which will, hopefully, hold my kneecaps in place throughout the day and ensure that they correctly track in the knee joint. Without the tape, my knees may become sore, and this will just add unnecessary discomfort. We gather together my wetsuit, goggles, flip-flops, bottles, and clothes to wear after the end of the race and head out of the hotel. Dude is excited to be coming with us, although he seems still sleepy as we leave the parking lot.

The race start is only ten minutes from the hotel, and even though it is only 5:00 a.m., there is a tremendous amount of activity as we approach the race site. Already, one of the race directors is announcing the temperature of the lake, still a cool 61 degrees. There are people everywhere milling about quickly with nervous energy. All the bikes have already been placed on the bike racks in transition. Twenty-five hundred bikes in neat rows, I can't even imagine the value of the combined amount; triathlon can certainly be an expensive business. I hear the soft whirring noise of the generators as they power the bright stadium lights and illuminate the bikes. I place my special-needs bags in their respective boxes. There is a special-needs bag for the bike and a separate one for the run. Each is given to you approximately halfway through each of these respective legs of the race and contains whatever you feel you may want at this point. Inside my bags are additional sports drink, gels, Vaseline, band-aids, and fresh socks. I check my bike. The tires are still firm, but I add additional air with my pump just because. Three women near to me ask to borrow my pump to do the same. It's a matter of just going through the checklist robotically, ensuring everything is just so. I fill up my aero-bottle with my special sports drink. My aero-bottle is located at the front of my bike between my aero-bars. This allows me to have easy access to my fluid without having to sit upright and lose my aerodynamic position.

Don and Dude watch patiently from the fence with the hoards of other family and friends. I make two more trips to the bathroom and then finally sit down to take in the moment. I'm excited to get started, and the nerves are now causing me to chatter nonstop with Don.

It is now 6:20 a.m. and time to put on my wetsuit. Even though I purchased a brand-new wetsuit this summer, I have chosen to wear my old wetsuit. I feel very comfortable in this suit, and I know it will get me through the 2.4 miles. As I carefully and slowly pull up each leg, however, I notice the tears, holes, and glue holding it together; perhaps this swim will be the last one for this wetsuit. I take my time and ensure that I do not create any new holes. At 6:30 a.m., I am ready to go. I kiss Don good-bye, and he wishes me luck. I remember a similar moment as I headed out for heart surgery eight months ago when he told me the surgery was just like an Ironman race…time to find out. I head down to the start line.

It is windy and cold for this time of year, and the forecast even calls for rain; this, however, is out of my control, and I know better than to worry about the conditions. It is the same for everyone else. It is still dark; the sun is trying to rise, but the clouds are blocking it, making the morning sunrise almost nonexistent. I stand on the edge of the lake amongst thousands of other participants. Everyone is excited. The professional triathletes are permitted to enter the lake before the amateurs (age-groupers). At 6:40 a.m., we are all allowed to jump into the lake. As I step forward and jump in, the cold water literally takes my breath away. I have so much adrenaline pumping around in my body that I struggle to breathe and almost have a small panic attack. I am a strong swimmer, I know that; I just need to stay calm and get a grip, so I stay still in the water for a few minutes, treading water and taking in the moment. Slowly, my breathing relaxes and I begin my warm-up.

It is still dark.

I swim some fast and slow strokes to try to raise my heart rate and body temperature, but it is hard to do in the cold water. All of a sudden, I hear the cannon fire; the professional race has begun. They start 10 minutes ahead of the age-groupers. I swim to the start line and ensure that I have plenty of space around me. I line up just to the right of the middle of the pack, second row back. I had spoken to a veteran Ironman Arizona participant yesterday who recommended this position based on my predicted swim time. "As a strong swimmer, you must line up at the front; otherwise, you will waste valuable time swimming over and around people much slower than you," he had advised me. All of a sudden, I see Dougal, my training partner, at the front also. I yell out to him, and we are both giddy and very surprised to see each other. I have swam with Dougal countless times over the summer in Lake Mead, and I know his swim pace is similar to mine, so I am comfortable with my positioning. We are treading water to keep warm.

It is still dark.

There is a hush and then quiet before the national anthem is sung. The race director gives the one-minute warning, and at this point, I start my watch and position my body forward onto my stomach with my arms stretched outwards to ensure I have plenty of space and get a good start.

And then it happens; the cannon fires loudly and we are off. My day of reckoning has begun.

The swim start in an Ironman event is always a mass start, which means everyone, all 2500 competitors, start together. Stronger swimmers should position themselves towards the front, and weaker swimmers towards the back. Regardless of the placing, however, the start is still a spectacle, and the splashing and frenzy that occur in those first few minutes is something quite amazing to see. My first few strokes are strong and fast; I am determined not to get caught up with the masses behind me, so I swim hard for approximately 200 meters. I am surprised that I don't get banged about too much by flailing arms and legs, and I bank this positive in my brain, as I may need to draw on the positives later in the day. The course is an elongated rectangle that totals 2.4 miles long. After a few minutes, I settle down and try to bilaterally breathe to ensure my stroke is smooth and my breathing under control. The lake is filled with runoff water, so it is very cloudy, and even when the sun starts to break through the clouds, I still cannot see my hands in front of me as they enter the water.

I feel strong, and I concentrate on my form; right, left, breathe, pull, catch, follow through, and rotate....all the phrases from my hours spent in the pool. I let other swimmers pass me; I am not going to increase my speed too soon. I know 2.4 miles will take me at least an hour, so I have many more minutes still ahead, and I need to pace myself according to my plan. Typically, this race has participants swimming into the sun for the first half of the course; however, today, there is very little sun to blind my sight, another positive. I keep the buoys on my left and count them off as I pass them all, until, all of a sudden, I see the big red turn buoy ahead. Great, that is my first left turn and the halfway point. There is some congestion near the buoy as swimmers jostle for position, not wanting to swim too far wide of the buoy unnecessarily. I stay strong and powerful, not letting anyone crowd me. Another hundred meters, and there is the second red turn buoy. another left turn, and now comes the back straight.

My plan is to slowly start to increase my speed on this section of the swim, but carefully, so as not to compromise my form. I start to increase my stroke rate without affecting my form; however, I notice a slight side stitch start to develop on the right side of my stomach. I slow the stroke back down and reach long to stretch out my torso. It works, and the stitch subsides. I lift my head up in front as I breathe in order to sight, and I see the last bridge about five hundred meters ahead of me. I still feel strong and decide that now is the time to pick up my pace. I increase my kick and quickly leave the person drafting behind me. I begin to pass other swimmers, one by one; I count them as I hunt them down. My adrenaline is still pumping, and I'm enjoying this moment. I'm delighted with my pacing strategy and proud that I had the discipline to execute it properly. I swim fast under the last bridge, and before I know it, the last red turn buoy is in front of me. I make my final left turn and head for the exit.

I'm still passing people in this final stretch. The water level in the lake is about a foot lower than is typical, and as a consequence, the metal steps out of the lake are not quite low enough into the water. There are six sets of steps, and I choose the fifth one on the right side, as I see a clear run into this exit line. I swim right up to the bottom step, then swiftly turn myself around onto my behind, then hoist myself up onto my feet. I had practiced this exit strategy the day before, and now I smile to myself and realize that just taking the time to practice this was time well spent. Other swimmers are scrambling and being helped by volunteers. I climb up the steps and head out to the swim finish over the timing chip mat. It bleeps as it records my swim time, one hour and three minutes; perfect, exactly where I wanted to be.

I pull out my earplugs and glance down at my watch. It shows a heart rate of 171 bpm. This is high but not unexpected at this point in the race; I know, however, that I will have to bring my heart rate down quickly once I'm on my bike. I jog towards a group of volunteers and then sit down on the ground while they aggressively strip off my wetsuit. They are quick, much quicker than I could be by myself, and I thank them for their help. My cap and goggles are still on my head, and I carry my wetsuit as I jog around the back of the transition site. I enter the section of gear bags and yell out my number, 2451. A volunteer grabs my bike gear bag and instructs me to run to the far entrance of the changing tent, the women's changing tent. All of a sudden, I hear, "Go, Elle!" I look to the left; there are Don and Dude cheering for me. I smile.

Two volunteers quickly usher me to a chair and pour out the contents of my bag on the floor; helmet on, socks on, shoes on, sunglasses on. In a matter of minutes, I am on my way. I yell, "Thank you!" back to the volunteers and see them carefully placing my wetsuit in the bag along with my goggles and swim cap. I run into the aisle between all the racked bikes. I know approximately where my bike is racked, as I had practiced this run the previous day. I head down the aisle marked 2400–2500. A volunteer is already head of me and unhooks my bike from the rack and hands it to me. I had strategically placed a lump of Vaseline under my seat (in case I needed some additional lubrication on the ride), and I wince, embarrassed as I notice the volunteer rub his hands on his shorts! I run with my bike out of the bike transition and then over another timing mat. This records my time from the swim exit to bike start, otherwise known as my T1 time, 5 minutes, 16 seconds. I carefully mount my bike, and off I go; 112 miles are ahead of me.

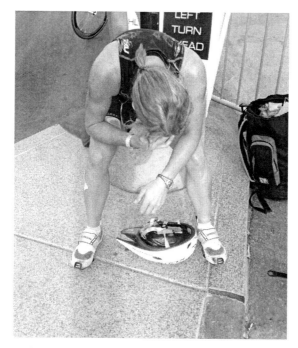

Post Silverman 2009, I am blind in my right eye

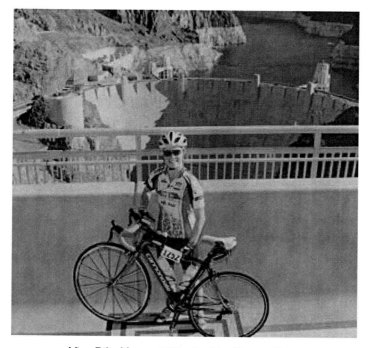

Viva Bike Vegas, 115 mile ride, Hoover Dam

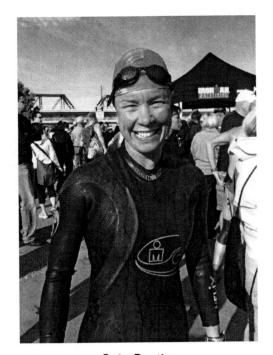

Swim Practice

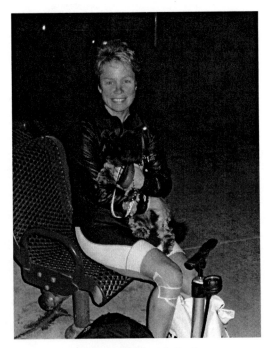

Race morning with Dude

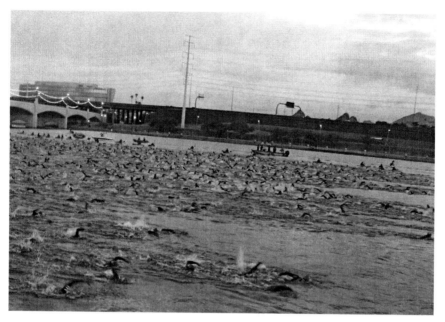

2500 Athletes

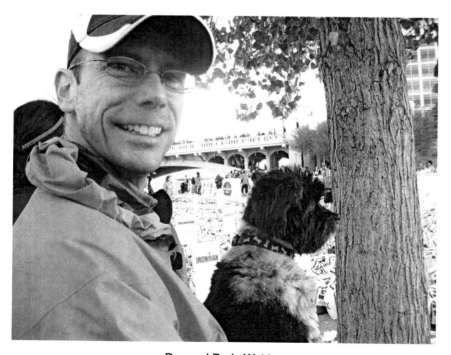

Don and Dude Waiting

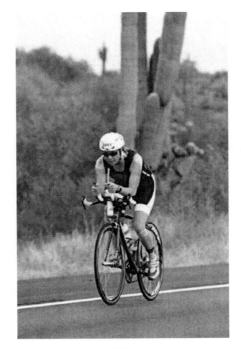

Riding

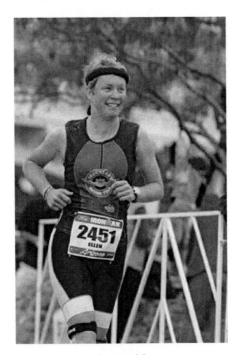

Loving It!

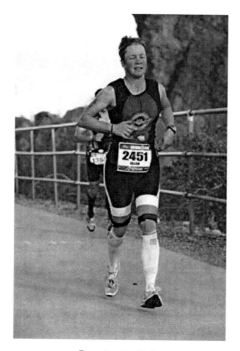

Running in Pain

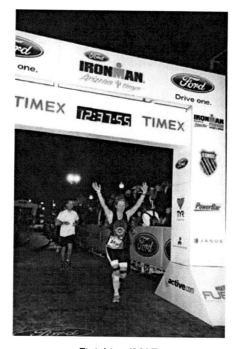

Finishing IMAZ

CHAPTER 15

Race Day: The Bike

November 2010

I t's cold; the wind is going to be a factor, but I know this is out of my control. What is in my control is my heart rate, and the first order of business is to lower it. I spin through the crowds in an easy gear, and, beat by beat, my heart rate lowers quickly. Once out of the race-site area, I get into my aero-position and settle in for the first section of the bike course. The course is a three-loop course, each loop identical, consisting of 37 miles. The first nine miles zigzag out of the town of Tempe in a northwesterly direction.

As I make the first few turns, I sit up out of my aero-bars and take the corners carefully; it is too early to be aggressive, and the last thing I need this early on is to crash. Because my swim time was relatively fast (I finished 271st out of 2500 participants), there are plenty of riders who pass me. I am not concerned, and, in fact, I am confident with my plan. The online training group that I had joined in October (Endurance Nation) has a well-thought-out and -tested approach to Ironman racing. I had listened to their strategy and, not having anything else to compare it with, decided to give it a go. One of their four keys to Ironman racing is that the race only truly begins at mile 18 of the run; therefore, an important strategy is to have a steady bike. They say to ride the pace that you should ride and not what you could ride, so that when you finish the bike portion, you still have plenty of energy to run the marathon. In fact, the Endurance Nation coaches preach that if you do the reverse of what everyone else is doing out there, you may well be in good shape. I am therefore happy that riders are passing me.

It is still cold, but I am warming up as my legs spin. I drink from my aero-bottle and feel good. My heart rate hovers around 140–150 bpm, perfect. I drink every 10 to 15 minutes. I have calculated out the exact amount of fluid, calories, sodium, and potassium that I will need to take in. What I didn't anticipate was that the temperatures would be cold enough such that my level of sweat is almost non existent. Still, I drink but soon realize that within just 15 miles, I will need a bathroom break.

An Ironman is a long day. Even for the pros it is a long race, but one in which every second counts. With this in mind, taking a bathroom break is often done while riding; yes, peeing on the bike is the norm for the pros. I contemplate this for a second or two but soon realize that this is a skill that clearly takes a lot of practice and today is not a good day for me to start practicing. I see the sign for the next aid station ahead and pull in to the side of the road. A volunteer kindly holds my bike while I visit the porta-potty. A few seconds later, I am on my way again, feeling happy with my decision to stop.

The wind speed is increasing as I ride onto the Beeline Highway, a straight road out for nine more miles with a slight 2% grade. The wind direction is behind me at this point, which is unusual for this time of year. I reach the turnaround point, and as I face the return portion of the highway, the headwind hits me like a bolt of lightning. Riders around me are equally surprised, and I hear shocked voices and the occasional expletive. I try not to be disheartened; I know I can ride in the low aerodynamic position and cut through the wind for a long time. I have trained in this position in Las Vegas. I ride on. Some riders pass me in groups; this is illegal, as riding as a pack provides shelter from the wind. If caught by the race marshals, the riders could receive a drafting penalty, which would mean having to sit in the penalty tent for four minutes before being allowed to continue the race. After three drafting penalties, the rider would be disqualified. I have never had a drafting penalty, and I don't intend to receive one on this race, even though the thought of sitting snugly behind another rider to avoid this headwind right now is attractive.

I see the 20-mile marker. Also on the sign are the numbers 57 and 94, indicating the number of miles achieved at that point on the second and third laps, respectively. I'm averaging approximately 17.5 miles per hour, a little slower than I know I could ride this course, but I have readjusted my goal because of the wind and now rain that is coming down. I hear a rider yell as the rain drives into us, "What the !@#$, this is meant to be the desert!" I smile to myself. There is no point getting upset at Mother Nature; she is out of my control.

My smile starts to fade within the next few minutes, however, as I start to feel a slight cramping in my stomach. Oh no, I had been praying that my ill-timed menstrual period would not cause these cramps, not today. But alas, the cramps continue and increase in strength, and very soon, I am officially in pain. It is worse as I lean into my aero-position and squeeze my bloated stomach. I allow myself one minute sitting upright every ten minutes. This seems to be sufficient to stop the cramping developing any further. The cramping doesn't subside, however. I focus on my box. This is Endurance Nation's second key to Ironman racing: focus on only those things immediately around you that you can control; don't think outside of your box, stay focused within in. My current box is the next five miles before I reach the end of the first lap. I hope I will see Don and my other friends, Amy and Bob, who have driven down from Las Vegas to Tempe just to see me race. That is all I need to stay positive.

In just a couple more miles, I can hear the crowds cheering for the riders. I sit up as I enter the turnaround point at the end of the first lap. I look around me but can see neither Don nor Amy or Bob. Oh well, time to turn around and get going on lap number 2. As I pull away from the crowds, I hear, "Go, Ellen, go!" I look to my left and see Dougal's wife, Kay, sitting on the side of the road cheering. I feel a warm glow within; at that moment I realize how powerful it is to see someone you know and know that they are cheering you on. Still no sign of Don, though. I head back out on familiar territory, zigzagging the first nine miles as I did approximately two hours and ten minutes ago. My stomach is no better, and the thought of a further four hours in this state is depressing. The wind is stronger still, and my morale is dropping.

Ironman racing typically delivers highs and lows to the competitors all day long. I know this is my first low point. It is all the more depressing because I didn't expect to feel in this much pain on the bike—the run, perhaps, but not the bike. I know I have to stay focused, stay in my box, and consider what I can do to get out of the low that I am slipping into.

As I turn north onto the Beeline Highway for the second time, the wind is at my back again and I thankfully hold onto this small positive. I continue to drink and take in more calories; I know I have to do this despite my stomach cramps, as I will never have the energy to run the marathon if I don't. I see the aid station that I stopped at on the last lap ahead and decide to make another pit stop, more to straighten up my body rather than because I urgently need to pee. Soon, I am on my way again, and the rest has given me some temporary relief from the cramps. I am in control of my attitude; I can control how I feel, and therefore, I will myself into a more positive state. It works, and before I know it, I am at the turnaround point. This marks the halfway point on the bike portion, 56 miles done. In just a few miles, there will be the optional stopping point for me to pick up my special-needs bag. I focus on this next milestone. As I enter the special-needs aid station, I search for my box along the side of the road and come to a stop next to number 2400–2500. Two volunteers help me swap out my empty bottles for my full bottles. I don't bother to take anything else from my bag. I haven't been able to eat the energy gels that I have in my storage pouch on my bike so have no need to replenish at this point.

As I set off again, the wind blows hard, and as a rider comes up on my left, he shouts across to me, "I'm not loving this wind." I look over to my left; by some amazing coincidence, I actually know this guy from my training days in Hawaii. His name is Brian, and I yell to him as he passes by. I don't think he recognizes me, but I explain to him who I am. I wish him well in the race, and he takes off ahead of me. I remember Brian being a stronger rider and runner than me, but I was a stronger swimmer, so it makes sense that he is only now just passing me on the bike. Seeing Brian gives me a mental boost, and I'm able to keep spinning and focused. I am soon hearing the crowds at the race site as I approach the end of my second lap. Again I search for familiar faces, but I don't see any. I presume Don is out running at this point; he has to run 14 miles today as part of his Las Vegas marathon training program. Perhaps I will see him on my third lap.

As I head out on lap number 3, I drop into my aero-position. My stomach screams at me, and I have no choice but to sit straight back up. I attempt to go low again two more times, but each time is unsuccessful, so I concede to ride this outward part of lap three sitting upright.

Fortunately for me, the wind is at my back for most of this portion, so I am not too disadvantaged. I hope that by the time I make the final turn, my stomach may have recovered a little to allow me to get into the aero-position again, which will be far more important as I tackle the headwind for the final time. My plan works, and even though riders around me are now sitting upright as they head into the wind, aching from being in the aero-position for so long, I am able to get low again and cut through the wind. My stomach behaves ever so slightly, or perhaps I am now just getting numb from the pain. I am now only nine miles from the end of the bike course.

I notice slower riders riding on the other side of the road heading out on their third or maybe just second lap. I don't envy them; I know now my end is in sight. I have seen several riders stopped at the side of the road fixing flat tires, and am grateful I have not had a flat tire to contend with; I feel very lucky. I make a right turn and begin the zigzag section in reverse. I am expecting the headwind to be a direct hit on the zig portions of the zigzag, and I am not wrong. Bam! Right at me. My pace slows to 13 miles per hour, and everyone around me is struggling and willing this to end. It is still cold, and the rain is now coming down hard. I make a left turn and get some relief; now it is only a crosswind, but a fierce one nonetheless.

I look up and see a sandstorm brewing to my left, and then within seconds, a strong gust literally blows me three feet across the road. I put on my brakes and steady my bike almost to a complete stop. Sand is all over me, and I can feel it on my face. I hear the riders behind me yell to others to slow down. I was the worst affected, but I feel strong and know that I have only a few miles left; not even a sandstorm will stop me now. I soldier on. I must look awful. I will myself to finish the bike portion strong. As I pull up to the turnaround point, this time I take the right lane and head to transition.

I feel for the riders starting their last lap; the wind is even stronger now. I ride through the transition area and get to the dismount line. A volunteer grabs my bike and tells me to run on into transition; I do as I'm told, so happy to be off the bike. Not only my stomach is happy to be upright, but my nether regions are too! I cross the timing mat again, 6 hours, 27 minutes, a little slower than I had hoped, but not significantly, and given the conditions both externally and internally, I am pleased overall. I was able to control my heart rate completely, which was the most important thing.

After the race, I read the results for my bike splits for each loop. They were almost exactly the same each loop, 17.5 miles per hour. I rode the bike portion exactly to plan, something that I am very proud of.

I jog through transition and hear my swim coach, Paul, yell at me. I turn around and see him with a huge proud smile on his face. I pick up my run gear bag and head back into the changing tent. I sit down and again have two volunteers help me get ready for the run portion. I put on my compression socks. (I have no idea whether they really help, but I've been training with them now for a few weeks and I like the way they feel, plus all the pros wear them!) One of the volunteers hands me the tampon that falls out from my bag and gives me a sympathetic smile. She explains where the porta-potty is, and I stop by before heading out on the run. I cross the timing mat again; my bike-to-run transition time is 4 minutes, 58 seconds. I am happy with this, given the pit stop I had to make. I hear the crowds shouting. They must be cold; they certainly look it. I thank the volunteers again and head out for the run. My first ever marathon awaits me, just 26.2 miles to go.

CHAPTER 16

Race Day: The Run

November 2010

I've never run a marathon before, and my longest training run was 20 miles. I was able to run this with an average of 10 minutes per mile. I had therefore calculated that my first six to eight miles should be slower than this pace, closer to an 11-minute mile. I set out slowly, just jogging. I look down at my watch, which gives my pace as well as my heart rate. I'm running at a pace of 10 minutes and 30 seconds per mile, a little faster than I probably should be going so early on, but I feel good and my heart rate is hovering around 140 bpm, so all is good.

Similarly to the bike course, the marathon is a three-loop course, each loop consisting of 8.7 miles around the lake. It isn't, however, a flat course, as there are three bridges that we have to climb up and over within each loop. The first stretch of the run is into the wind, but I'm not too worried by this; at least it will keep my body temperature low and ensure I don't overheat. At the first mile marker, I see two women spectators on the right-hand side of the pathway, clapping and cheering each runner as they go by. I feel goose bumps down my spine. For the first time, I allow myself to consider that I will be an Ironman in a few hours. Quickly, I stop my mind wandering and bring my thoughts back to my new box. I know the race doesn't really begin until mile 18, and I need to stay in control until that point.

As recommended by Endurance Nation and also as practiced in my training runs, I walk for 30 steps at the end of each aid station; this gives me something to look forward to each mile and also gives me some brief recovery time and opportunity to properly take in fluid. I try the new sports drink that the race volunteers offer; the fruit punch flavor is a welcome break from the lemonade I drank on the bike.

The cramping returns shortly after mile 2, and my stomach bloats; it hurts to suck it in, and it hurts to run. I have 24 miles to go, and the thought of another four hours of pain is hard to comprehend. I try to focus and think of how to get ahead of the pain and mentally will it away. Perhaps if I take another bathroom break, I will be able to crouch over and give my stomach some temporary relief. At the next aid station, I try this, and the pain subsides for just a few minutes before returning again and remaining as a dull ache. I know I have to think of other things to take my mind off the pain, and so I begin to think about all that I have accomplished this year. I relive the heart surgery, the pain during those first few days as I lay in my hospital bed, the first steps I took as I walked around the hospital ward holding Don's arm for support, the pain as the tubes were removed from my neck and chest, and the constant nausea for the days following surgery. This not only takes my mind off my aching stomach but also gives me renewed strength.

Aid stations on the run course are strategically positioned at approximate one-mile intervals. It is reassuring to know that you are only ever a matter of minutes away from food, fluid, and a bathroom. Each aid station is manned with dozens of kind and excited volunteers. Some of the aid stations are decorated with a theme and the volunteers are dressed in costumes to add a little light entertainment for the athletes. I am very thankful to all the volunteers.

At mile 7, I hear my name screamed loudly, and I look ahead to see Don jumping up and down with excitement. I yell back and smile a smile as big as I can muster; this is a battle I will not lose, I will finish. I yell to Don that I'm feeling great, even though I'm not, in the hope that my brain will trick my stomach. I know that I control how I feel.

I hear the crowds as I run along the path at the side of the lake. I am nearing the race site and will soon begin my second loop. Only 16 more miles to go, I know I can do this. The crowds are amazing, and I can hear them cheering some of the pros who are finishing at this time. It is mentally tough knowing I have two more loops to go, but I also feel invigorated from the noise and excitement.

Before I know it, I'm beginning my second lap and soon pass the two women sitting on their foldaway chairs that I had seen an hour and forty minutes ago. They cheer loudly again and shout words of encouragement as I pass them for the second time. The sun is now starting to set, and I know they must be cold. As I cross over the bridge, I start to run alongside a younger female athlete. All athletes have their age printed on their calf, and I can see she is only 25 years old. She is very small and looks cold, but we chat and confirm that this is the first Ironman for each of us. We run a similar pace until the next aid station and then we separate as I adopt my 30 walking paces at the end of the station. I decide to try something different at this aid station, and the thought of Coke is appealing to me; perhaps the bubbles will calm my stomach a little. This was a bad plan. Within minutes of taking in the Coke, I'm nauseated. In fact, it is the worst I have felt so far, and I have to run with a little bend at the waist to ease the pressure on my poor bloated stomach.

One more mile, keep putting one foot in front of the other, you are strong, you have endured much worse than this.

The third key that Endurance Nation preaches is to know and to rehearse your "one thing," the "one thing" that is the reason you are doing the Ironman, the reason why you have invested so many hours of training and the reason why you are still putting one foot in front of the other. I had thought about my "one thing," and it was pretty simple: for me. The reason I wanted to be an Ironman was to prove to myself that nothing is impossible and that nothing is going to derail my dream, not even heart surgery. At mile 11, I focus on my one thing.

I hear my name again. I look around and see Don again, this time with my friends Bob and Amy. They are all cheering and jumping up and down. "Elle, you look amazing; you are gorgeous!" And then I hear another spectator echo Don's words and yell, "Yes, you do!" That was enough to get me through the next two miles to the halfway point and then to the special-needs station. I had forgotten to pack my magic wand, so I knew there was nothing in my bag that would magically cure my stomach pains, but even so, I am excited just to get my bag and look inside and confirm that indeed there is nothing I actually need at this time. I have plenty of fluid and gels and don't need new socks or a long-sleeved tee shirt; I'm not cold even though the sun is now on its way down.

Only a half marathon to go; I know I will now finish, even if I have to walk the last few miles. I know I will finish within the 17-hour deadline; this realization spurs me on, and I am able to temporarily forget the pain for the next few miles. Almost at the end of lap 2 now, I again can hear the crowds cheering at the race site. I'm starting to imagine crossing the finish line, and my eyes start to well up. I quickly stop the thoughts; I still have another loop to go, and approximately nine more miles stand between me and the finish.

I start the final loop. It is now dark, and volunteers are giving out luminous bracelets for the participants. The bracelets don't provide any light for you to see your footing, but they do allow others to see you. I don't take one, as I figure the run course is mostly on a pathway and the roads are closed to the traffic. At mile 18, I expect my legs to drop off or for something else to happen because I had been warned several times that at mile 18, the wall can hit and the race really begins. Hours can be lost in these last eight miles if you have to spend more time walking than running. Surprisingly, my legs stay intact. My stomach even starts to feel a little better, and if anything, I feel a little stronger at mile 18. Success! Perhaps my pacing wasn't too bad after all. I look down at my watch and see my pace has slowed to an 11-minute mile while I'm running, but I know that my average pace will be slower, given the four bathroom breaks I've taken on the run. Still, I am pleased with how I feel at this point and that my heart rate is still only 140 bpm. I start to look forward to the mile markers. Number 19 comes and goes, and I don't look back. Then I see Don again one more time. He runs with me for about 100 meters but is worried that him running next to me may be classified as outside assistance, so he tells me he will see me at the finish line, that I look fantastic, and that he is so very proud of me. I smile and hold back the tears; I still have six miles to go.

As I run on, I decide that now that I have less than six miles to go, I will not stop at all, not even at the aid stations; I just want to get to the finish line as soon as possible, and even a very slow jog is faster than a walk. I look at my run split time so far and calculate that I can run a sub–five-hour marathon if I just focus and keep going; this becomes my new box. I pass countless people in those last five miles. Many of them are walking now; perhaps they are on lap 3 or maybe still on lap 2. They cheer as I jog past them. "Way to finish strong!" I hear someone say.

The final key from the Endurance Nation coaches is that the race is about execution and not fitness. As I run past athletes who can do no more than walk, I am proud that I have executed my race according to my plan. I still have the energy to jog these last few miles. Fitness alone cannot get you through an Ironman.

I get to mile 21. This is new territory for me. I smile, knowing that every step for me is a Charnley world record from here and that I am only minutes away from victory.

The soles of my feet hurt. They are screaming at me to stop, but I will not stop; I cannot stop. My heart is beating faster now, and once again, the adrenaline is pumping. I am on the other side of the lake, and I look across and see the lights surrounding the finish area. I can also hear the crowds as the wind carries their cheers across to me. I have two miles to go, up and over the bridge, then the home stretch. Keep moving, left, right, left, right. I run onto the bridge and up the slight slope, across, and down the other side. Now I am on the home stretch, and I pass the 25-mile mark. Tears roll down my cheeks. I allow them to continue until I can't breathe anymore. Just a few more minutes. I pass the final aid station and thank the volunteers as I glide through. I feel like I'm flying, but in reality, I know I'm only shuffling.

I make the final turn to the left and start the 100 meters down the finishing chute. The crowd is going wild; it is utterly amazing: bright lights, screams, and waving hands, people high-fiving me as I run the final few meters. I hear Don scream to my left, and I wave, with tears flowing down my cheeks. I look up at the finish clock and see my finish time of 12 hours and 37 minutes, faster than my wildest dreams. I cross the finish line and raise my arms in the air. Tears roll down my face as I hear my name on the loudspeaker. "Ellen Charnley, you are an Ironman!"   Eight months, almost to the day since my open-heart surgery, I have never felt more alive.

Epilogue

I have never experienced such a sense of achievement. It is hard to describe. I am overwhelmed still weeks after the race. My adrenaline levels have slowly lowered, but I still wake up early each morning, pinch myself, and ask Don if I really am an Ironman. There has been a constant stream of congratulatory messages and phone calls. I am flattered and shocked that some of my friends have shared a tear of joy with me these past few days. Some have no idea what becoming an Ironman really entails, but others, fellow Ironmen, smile and nod to show their admiration. My medical team at the Cleveland Clinic expressed their amazement and also showed how proud they were by inviting me to run alongside the Robotic Cardiac Surgeon Team at the 2011 Cleveland Marathon next May. I will be honored to run alongside them next spring.

There are currently only 25 official Ironman events in the world. Ten of these are in North America, and the rest span the globe, across Asia, Europe, Australia, Africa, and South America. At each event, anywhere from 1500 to 2500 athletes complete the event. This is a tiny percentage of the world's population; therefore, becoming part of this elite club is something very special. It is not uncommon to parade an M-dot tattoo as evidence of membership to this special cult.

Just five days after the race, I received my M-dot tattoo, something that I have dreamed about for years. My tattoo contains not only the M-dot trademark but also a small mended heart next to it. This has marked the end of my extraordinary Ironman journey.

Twenty ten has been an amazing year in which I have experienced both the lowest and highest points of my life. Without the lows, I doubt that the highs would have felt so sweet. My journey has been very real, and I wouldn't change any part of it. I feel blessed to have experienced and lived through it all. I'm looking forward to many years ahead, and one thing is certain: I will continue to live my life to the fullest.

CPSIA information can be obtained at www.ICGtesting.com
Printed in the USA
236083LV00001B/5/P